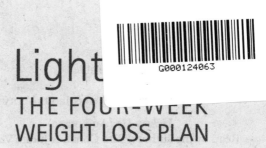

Light
THE FOUR-WEEK
WEIGHT LOSS PLAN

Also available

Lighten Up – Pete Cohen & Judith Verity

Lighten Up (Audiotape)
Read by the authors, Pete Cohen & Judith Verity

Lighten Up

THE FOUR-WEEK
WEIGHT LOSS PLAN

Pete Cohen and Judith Verity

ARROW

5 7 9 10 8 6

Arrow Books
20 Vauxhall Bridge Road
London SW1V 2SA

Arrow Books is part of the Penguin Random House group of companies
whose addresses can be found at global.penguinrandomhouse.com

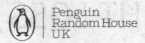

Penguin
Random House
UK

First published in the United Kingdom in 2003 by Arrow Books

www.penguin.co.uk

A CIP catalogue record for this book is available
from the British Library

ISBN 978 0 09 944664 4

Design & make up by Roger Walker

Penguin Random House is committed to a sustainable future for
our business, our readers and our planet. This book is made from
Forest Stewardship Council® certified paper.

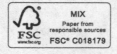

MIX
Paper from
responsible sources
FSC® C018179

Printed and bound in Great Britain by Clays Ltd, St Ives plc

Contents

Introduction

Welcome to Lighten Up, the slimming programme that can help you become slimmer, healthier and fitter. Hundreds of diets or exercise programmes claim to make a lasting difference, but Lighten Up really does: the average long-term success rate for a slimming programme is only 5%, but nearly 70% of people who've followed the Lighten Up programme have not only *become* slimmer but *stayed* slimmer.*

So why is Lighten Up different? Well it's different because it's the product of years of experience working with people just like you. It's not an abstract idea, it's a straightforward response to the problems encountered by real people in the real world.

The first elements of the Lighten Up programme started to come together back in the 1980s when Pete Cohen became concerned about how to help people who wanted to lose weight. At the time he was working as a personal trainer so he started, naturally enough, with exercise. When he found that exercise alone didn't work he tried putting together balanced, varied nutritional programmes for his clients. But however desperate people say they are, desperation alone is never enough to make them stick to drastic exercise routines and diet sheets.

Eventually he decided that motivation might be the missing ingredient. He introduced his slimming clients to some of the motivational sports psychology techniques he used with ath-

* Based on a study conducted by Lighten Up.

letes, and, at last, he started to see results. Not only were his clients getting slimmer, fitter and healthier, they were staying that way. They were feeling good about themselves. They were enjoying a more active lifestyle – and they were eating when they were hungry and not feeling guilty about it.

Which is how Lighten Up began.

The Lighten Up Success Formula

When Pete met health and fitness writer Judith Verity they decided to start Lighten Up. They began with eight-week courses, teaching people how to take control of their eating – and their lives – and then, a few years later, they wrote a book about it called *Lighten Up*. The book was a great success, but as demand for the courses increased they discovered that lots of people wanted a quicker way to Lighten Up so they developed a new, more intensive, four-week course to meet that demand.

This book will take you, step by step, through the new fast-track, four-week course. You'll be using the amazingly success-ful ideas and techniques they've perfected with the help of thousands of slimmers who have tried and tested them through their real life experience of Lightening Up.

So what is Lighten Up?

We don't like the word 'diet' because diets tend to be associated with deprivation, with stress and – often – with failure. There's always the implication that a diet is something you only do for a while – but if it's only ever temporary, you're never going to make a long-term change to your life, are you?

Isn't a long-term transformation what you want? Don't you want to become slimmer and healthier forever, not just for that holiday or that special party? Lighten Up is all about learning a new way of eating – and living: it's something that allows you to get on with your life and sets you free from the endless cycle of dieting and putting on weight again. Lighten Up isn't a diet. So what is it?

- It's not just about short-term weight loss. It's about being permanently slimmer, fitter, healthier and happier.

- It's holistic. We want you to work with your body, eat when you're hungry, and treat yourself very well.

- Lighten Up empowers you to make your own decisions and lifestyle choices. From now on you can take control of the size and shape you're in.

- Lighten Up is the first slimming system to cover all three essential steps to slimness:

  > Motivation
  >
  > Eating
  >
  > Exercise

Lighten Up isn't simply about a quick fix. It's a permanent lifestyle change.

How to Read the Book

Are we kidding? No. Because Lighten Up is a four-week programme, it's important that you work your way through it *in chronological order*.

- Begin by reading through the first two chapters, and then take the rest one day at a time. The structure of the rest of the book makes it easy to follow as it provides you, day by day, with new ideas, new goals and – most importantly – the support and encouragement you need. You'll find a list of challenges at the beginning of each day, and they're then highlighted in the text so it's easy to see exactly what you're focusing on.

- The first thing you need to do is decide when you want to start. Most people go for a Monday – it seems somehow logical – but, although any day is fine, you do need to make a decision.

- The programme is then divided into four weeks, each of which is broken down into seven days, which you work through one at a time. There's a short 'Starter' section just before Day One of each week to get you in the right frame of mind – you can either read this the night before you begin, or run through it first thing on Day One. It's up to you.

- Then, the ideal way to do the programme is to put aside fifteen minutes or so each morning to read through and digest each new chapter at the beginning of the day, but of course not everyone has a daily schedule that allows for that – or you might not be a morning person! If you're not, just put aside a little more time on the Sunday night to read through the whole week, then you can just flick through and do a quick five-minute recap at the beginning of each day.

- However you decide to do it, it's crucial that you take it day by day and make sure you do at least read through your daily challenges first thing – it's only ten to fifteen minutes a day (that's only just over an hour for the whole week) so it's really worth finding the time to fit it into your daily schedule. Apart from anything else, it's a brilliant way to keep yourself focused – if you start the day feeling positive and concentrating on the new slim you, aren't you less likely to reach for that mid-morning bag of crisps?

- As you read through the book, you'll find shaded Challenge boxes giving instructions. These are key to making Lighten Up work for you. It might be tempting to skip past them, but please do stop and do whatever they ask. However trivial it seems it will make a big difference!

- Chapter 4 is about the rest of your life, so save that one until you've finished the four-week course.

- Chapters 6 and 7 are about exercise and food and you can dip into them whenever you want.

- If at any time you feel unsure of yourself, or you have a bit of a lapse, don't worry! Just go back to the last day on which you felt comfortable, and start again there.

One last thought . . .

Because Lighten Up is about eating and exercise, please take advice if you have any medical concerns. Before you start the programme, please consult your doctor if:

- you have not exercised for some time or you have any medical problems

- you are diabetic or you have any other medical condition which may affect your eating.

Chapter 1

Lighten Up

The Ultimate Diet

I wonder why you picked up this book, out of the thousands of slimming books you might have chosen. Is it the very first time you've thought about being slimmer? If so, congratulations! Following the Lighten Up Four-Week Programme means never having to worry about your weight again because, for the vast majority of people, slim, fit and healthy is the natural way to be.

However, it's much more likely that you chose *Lighten Up* because you've tried to lose weight before and you've heard that Lighten Up was different.

'I've tried everything . . .'

'I've tried everything' is often one of the first things people say when they sign up for one of our courses. In fact there are more than 300,000 diets in the world so nobody's actually followed every one – but even if you've only tried a few of them, we're happy to be your last resort.

And I know that for most of you we *will* be the last resort, because, as I've already mentioned, Lighten Up has a 67% success rate compared to 5% for other slimming programmes.*
Once you've Lightened Up, the chances are that your weight won't be on your mind – or on your waist – any more.

* Based on a study conducted by Lighten Up.

Lighten Up is different

Why is Lighten Up different from all those other slimming methods? It's simply because most of the others are incomplete. They don't give you all the tools you need to keep the weight off permanently. Most of them are simply diets; although of course sticking to a very strict diet will make you lose weight for the duration of the diet, dieting alone is unlikely to help you lose weight permanently. In fact, in the long term, it's more likely to make you gain weight than lose it – 95% of dieters fail to lose weight permanently* and many of them, over time, will gain more than they lost. If you're not convinced by the statistics, have a look at the table below and see how many of the statements you agree with:

(DO THIS NOW!)

What has dieting done for you?	Agree	Disagree
Dieting makes me think more about food than I usually do		
Dieting stops me eating when I'm hungry		
Dieting takes away the pleasure of eating		
Dieting takes the fun out of socialising		
Dieting is addictive		

Dieting doesn't work and it isn't fun. So why do it?

But as you probably know by now, Lighten Up isn't a diet at all, so you can relax and let go of your past dieting disasters. This is different.

* A survey carried out by *Psychology Today* and quoted in *Cover* magazine, January 1998.

Shock Tactics

Victoria sat in her first Lighten Up group looking sceptical: 'I wouldn't be here,' she said, 'if I hadn't already tried everything else. In fact, I'd given up. Then my daughter decided to get married and I went to help her buy a wedding dress. The changing rooms were all mirrors and I was pinning up the hem of her dress when I looked up and saw this fat, middle-aged woman. I thought it was the assistant. Then I realised it was me. I said to my daughter, "Do I really look that bad?" and I could see how embarrassed she was. It was the pause before she lied to me that made me come here.'

A lot of people are shocked into Lightening Up by a traumatic Scrooge experience. Remember the story of Scrooge in *A Christmas Carol*? Over the years, Scrooge gradually becomes meaner and more miserable, but it's not until he's confronted by the awful picture of how much worse things can still get, that he finally decides to change.

Do you think you might have got so used to the way you are that you've almost given up? If so, there's no need to wait for an unexpected sighting in a changing room mirror, or an embarrassing moment when you try on last year's swimsuit, or even a tactless comment from a friend or enemy. You can look into your own Future Mirror right now and give yourself that motivational boost you need to get you started.

(DO THIS NOW!)

The Future You Don't Want

Ask yourself these questions and think carefully about the answers you get.

Of course, everybody's different, but if *you* go on living the way you are now, can you imagine what sort of shape you'll be in, six months or a year from now? Two years from now? Or even five years from now? ➡

Will you be even bigger than you are at present? Will you be less healthy perhaps? Less active? Less attractive? What sort of clothes will you be wearing? What kind of life will you lead? Does it matter?

The easiest thing you can do is nothing. So imagine that your plan of action continues to be a plan of inaction.

You're going to carry on eating the 'wrong' things, exercising too little, craving sugar like an addict and treating your body like a bin. Whatever it is you've done over the past months and years that has got you into the shape you're in right now, you're going to go right on doing it. After all, you're good at it by now, aren't you? You've practised weighing yourself every morning and beating yourself up. You've practised skipping breakfast and over-compensating with elevenses. You've practised cheering yourself up with chocolate...

If this sounds a bit depressing, that's good. Being really fed up with the way things are means you've finally had enough!

You could be ready to make those lasting changes. At last. All you have to do is spend a few minutes imagining how much *worse* things could get if you *don't* make those changes.

That's enough negative thinking for now – after all, the future you've just been looking at hasn't yet happened. But I hope the Scrooge exercise will have strengthened your determination to succeed this time, so we can get ready to start the slimming process.

Motivation, Eating and Exercise

If you've tried in the past to lose weight by any method that didn't involve changes in *all three* of these areas of your life (just by dieting perhaps, or just by joining a gym), you already know that it's unlikely to work forever. So, every day for the next four weeks, you'll be tackling *all three* of these, looking at your motivation as well as your eating and exercise habits.

Motivation – Slimming from the Head Down

Why do we start with Motivation? I know motivational thinking can seem a bit vague – I'm sure some of you are reading this and worrying that it's going to be terribly airy-fairy and abstract – but thousands of sceptics have tried it and made a long-term difference to their lives. It works, because, until you change the way you think about yourself and food, you won't be able to make the changes you want to make to your eating and exercise patterns. It's actually very simple, and it's why Lighten Up is sometimes called slimming from the head down.

The Lighten Up collection of tried and tested motivational techniques includes a well-known method used by athletes to help them achieve their goals and improve their performance. It is of course Visualisation, a tool that's both simple and effective. In fact, it's so obvious and so low tech that a lot of people won't even try it. And some reject it because it isn't difficult enough (after all, slimming's meant to be really, really hard). Others dismiss it because they've decided, in advance, that it's going to be too hard: that it won't work for them.

But remember the exercise you did just now, when you thought about what would happen if you didn't take action? The Future You Don't Want, or the Scrooge exercise as we call it. Well, that was Visualisation. The only difference between that particular Visualisation and the rest of the Lighten Up programme is that the Scrooge exercise can be rather negative – and quite upsetting for some people.

So why do we start off with it? Well, for one thing, it's much easier to get people to visualise things going wrong. Many of us are fixated on disaster scenarios – that's why we watch soap operas and scary films. We're always ready to see all the potential problems in our own lives too – that's why many people get depressed and anxious – but if you can picture things going wrong, it just proves that you can picture things. So from now on we're going to get you to picture them going right.

The second reason we start off with the Scrooge exercise is that it's such a powerful way to get you fired up for change and move you away from what you don't want.

So run through that Future You Don't Want scenario once more if you need an extra boost and then leave it behind you. From now on *positive thinking rules*. In fact, positive thinking is one of the most important Lighten Up principles.

Sounding slim

Thinking positive means talking positive as well – especially when you're talking to yourself.

(DO THIS NOW!)

Talking To Yourself

'I ought to lose weight.'

Not very motivational, is it? But I've talked to thousands of slimmers over the years and most of them are constantly talking to themselves about the weight they want to lose and picturing themselves as overweight people. If you think of yourself as overweight, it's going to seem natural for you to live like an overweight person.

'I must stop eating chocolate.'

Doesn't that make you feel like heading down to the shops for one last jumbo-size version of your favourite chocolate bar? And maybe a bag of fun size ones for later, since it's the last day you'll ever eat chocolate again? ▷

Say this to yourself instead:

'I'm going to be slimmer.'
'I'm getting slimmer.'
'I'm feeling slimmer.'
'I am slimmer, fitter and healthier.'

and

'I'm eating healthy food.'
'I'm drinking plenty of water.'
'I'm eating slowly.'
'I'm enjoying more exercise.'

From now on I want you to spend as much time listening to yourself as you spend at the moment listening to other people. Listen to what you say when you talk to yourself. Experiment with the words you use. Which ones motivate you?

Seeing Slim

Whether you believe me or not, you are amazing. Your body and brain are the most complex, high tech pieces of equipment and the most powerful computer you will ever own. But most people find it quite hard to really believe how amazing they are, so let's start with something easier.

(DO THIS NOW!)

Exercise Your Imagination

If I ask you to recall your last holiday, you're probably already thinking about the sea, the sand, the snow, the scenery, the bars and restaurants, the clothes you wore and the souvenirs you brought back. You could probably describe it in quite a bit of detail.

And if I asked you to describe your next holiday, the one you're planning, or the one you wish you could take, I bet you could describe that almost as clearly – in spite of the fact that you haven't been there and done it yet.

Imagination simply means 'making images'. Your brain doesn't know or care whether they are images of things you've done or images of things you'd like to do. Do you see where this is leading?

You can start, right now, to make this slimming process very easy for yourself by flexing your imagination muscles as often as possible.

Get into the habit of thinking about what it will be like when you succeed. When you reach your goal and become slimmer, more active, more confident and free at last from the tyranny of food.

Eating

What about the other two parts of Lighten Up: Eating and Exercise? Aren't they equally important? Well, of course they are – but we start with the motivational stuff because that's what makes the rest of it easy. And this is going to be easier than you can imagine.

Getting the right food inside you is vital, and the first step is to think about it carefully, because what you eat is determined by what you think.

'Engage your brain before opening your mouth.' If you've heard that saying and thought it only applied to thinking before you speak, think again. Thinking before you eat is a good idea too, especially if you want to be slim and healthy. Why? Because:

- If you think you're a fat person, you'll eat like one.

- If you think you want chocolate and you're given a diet sheet that's all about salad, you'll soon abandon it.

- If you're confused by the constant barrage of contradictory advice about what's bad for you and what isn't, you may give up and eat what everybody else does (even if it's not right for you).

Eating is one of life's great pleasures and it's also essential. So we'll be talking about eating a wide variety of healthy food with lots of fresh fruit and vegetables and drinking plenty of water. We'll be helping you beat your cravings, loosen the hold that certain foods may have over you, and become more aware of what your body needs. And most important of all, we'll be getting rid of the guilt and suggesting you start *enjoying your meals* even more.

Exercise

Exercise may be last on the list, but it's probably the most important factor in weight control. Although people in the developed world eat fewer calories than fifty years ago, we are gaining weight because we take so little exercise. The people who succeed in losing weight permanently are the ones who adopt a more active lifestyle.

But for some people, exercise is the scariest bit of all. 'I've done plenty of diets,' said Lizzy, 'and I hated them all – well, no, that's not quite true. The vodka diet was fun while it lasted. But I can tell you I haven't exercised since I wasn't chosen for the hockey team at school and I don't intend to start now.'

'But you don't mind walking, do you?' I said. (I'd walked up from the station with her and it was just over a mile.) 'Walking doesn't count,' she said. 'Everybody walks.'

Well, actually, a lot of people don't walk any more, but I knew what she meant. A lot of people think that exercise only keeps you slim if it makes you miserable and, even better, if it hurts as well.

Of course, that's rubbish. Done in the right way, exercise doesn't hurt – if it does, then you're trying to work at too high a level or doing the wrong kind of exercise for you. Much as you might not believe it now - and I don't expect you to take my word for it – exercise will make you feel more relaxed and comfortable in yourself. Even gentle exercise, once it's part of your daily routine, will make you feel better, give you more energy, help regulate your appetite and help you sleep well at night.

I'll be giving you more information over the next four weeks and if you want, you can dip into Chapters 5 and 6 which are all about exercise. For now, however, all you need to remember is this: Lighten Up isn't about extreme exercise or punishing fitness regimes, but it is about getting you moving – and you simply *can't* lose weight forever unless you're prepared to do that.

The Lighten Up Fat Burning Pyramid

The Lighten Up Fitness Programme is called the Fat Burning Pyramid and over the next four weeks you'll be gradually building your Fat Burning Pyramid, starting from the bottom. You'll be doing this according to your age, fitness and state of health so remember, the Lighten Up rule for fat burning fitness is that you always stay within your pleasure zone.

If you haven't enjoyed exercise in the past, and you've categorised yourself as a couch potato you may find it hard to imagine enjoying a more active lifestyle. Or perhaps you have health or mobility problems and you're getting panicky thoughts: 'If this involves drastic exercise it isn't for me…'

Relax. This programme is about getting more out of life and having fun. That's why it's called Lighten Up. We'll be helping you discover how you might lead a more active life based on the pleasure principle. After all, if you don't enjoy what you do, you aren't going to do it for very long.

Feel Good Fitness
30–60 minutes more strenuous exercise
every other day. Includes any form of fairly
concentrated exercise – things like:
    Aerobics
    Jogging
    Fast swimming

Fat Jar Fitness*
15 minutes of brisk activity, several
times a day. For example:
    Walking
    Housework
    Gardening
    Cycling
    Playing games with children

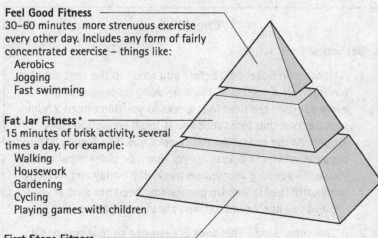

First Steps Fitness
Simple exercises that are a good base to your exercise programme

* Don't worry – we'll explain this on page 57

*If you have a medical condition that affects your breathing,
circulation or mobility, it is advisable to see your doctor before
starting any new exercise or activity.*

Checklist

Get yourself:

1. A Lighten Up Notebook. Before you go on to the next chapter, buy yourself a notebook. You'll be using up several pages every day over the next four weeks so you don't need a huge one. Get one that looks nice and is small enough to carry around. At the end of the four weeks, you'll be buying a Diary because, when the course is over, you'll be planning ahead for yourself – keeping yourself on track, day by day and week by week until the Lighten Up programme becomes part of your life and you don't need to think about it any more.

2. A Slimming Buddy. This book is designed so that you *can* go solo for the next four weeks if you prefer it that way, but if you'd like to work through the programme with a friend or relative you'll find it can be a lot of fun.

Chapter 2
Getting Started

FIRST:

- *Allow a bit of time to read this chapter. It's best to read it through at home, because there are some things you will probably want to do straight away.*

- *You'll also need that Notebook I mentioned, so have it to hand before you start reading.*

The Struggle to be Slim

Now that I've explained the three basic principles behind the Lighten Up programme, we're almost ready to start Day One. But before we do, there's some practical preparation that will give you a much better chance of success.

It's Time To Stop Being a Loser

To quote Victoria again: 'I've been fighting this for so long . . . it's just a constant battle, I'm always thinking about what I can't eat. It's a struggle – and every so often I lose it and give up and then I have to start all over again.'

You want to be slim, but you know it's a jungle out there. Food is everywhere. It's on the street, on the TV and in the newspapers and magazines. When life goes wrong – or even when it's just plain boring – it often seems that the easiest thing you can do is give in and eat, whether you're hungry or not.

And sometimes, just when you think you're getting it right, life sneaks up and knocks you off your feet. You know it's true. It's happened often enough before, hasn't it? You eat salad for a couple of days – then you lose the plot and have a doughnut or some croissants. After that, it's all downhill. Until the next diet.

Not any more. That was then. This time you're fighting back.

Getting Ready to Win the Battle

Yes, I know you think you've fought this battle before, and last time you got miserable, you got hungry, you got depressed – and ultimately of course you got a takeaway and put out the white flag till you felt strong enough to fight another day. Well, this time it's different. This time, you won't be the one who's hurting. It's going to be your old lifestyle and your old eating habits which bite the dust. Because this time you're going to set yourself up for success.

Setting Up Your Slimming Space

The Slimming Campaign Headquarters

First of all, you're going to give yourself a clear head start by creating a pressure-free zone where you'll have space to establish your new lifestyle, and the obvious place to set up your slimming campaign headquarters is your own home.

The Kitchen

The kitchen, of course, is clearly the place to start. This is where so many of us come to grief at midnight, or breakfast time, or when we get in from work. If you're too tired to do anything, the easiest thing to do is eat. After all, where do you go when you feel the first pangs of boredom, tension or loneliness? For most of us, it's the fridge. When we're too hungry to prepare a meal, the easiest snacks are often the sweetest. If we're anxious or depressed, we're much more likely to reach for the comfort food we've used to cheer ourselves up ever since we were children.

I'm not going to ask you to clear your kitchen out and fill the fridge with salad – Lighten Up is about making choices, not eliminating them – but taking a good hard look at your kitchen will give you a good idea of what your current habits and weaknesses are.

DO THIS NOW!

The Un–Shopping List

The diagram on page 22 is the Lighten Up Food Profile diagram, and it's absolutely central to the eating part of the Four-Week Plan.

Take a look at the two circles and then spend ten minutes checking off the contents of your fridge, freezer and store cupboards. Make it rough and ready. Put one cross for every item, regardless of size, and if you aren't sure about what category everything falls into just look at Chapter 7.

When you've finished, have a look at the two circles. What do you see? Chances are, you've put more crosses in Foods To Limit than Foods To Focus On.

What you do now is up to you. If you want, you can make the decision now to eliminate some of the Foods To Limit by having a clear-out. Or you can just put them in a separate cupboard so you're not confronted with them every time you go into the kitchen.

Or just think about this: next time you run out, do you need to replace them?

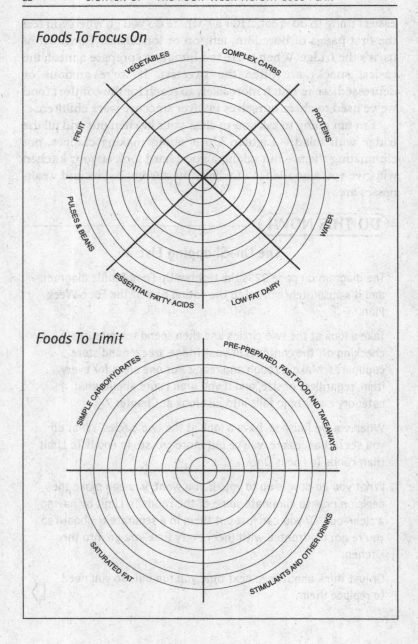

Foods To Focus On

VEGETABLES
COMPLEX CARBS
FRUIT
PROTEINS
PULSES & BEANS
WATER
ESSENTIAL FATTY ACIDS
LOW FAT DAIRY

Foods To Limit

SIMPLE CARBOHYDRATES
PRE-PREPARED, FAST FOOD AND TAKEAWAYS
SATURATED FAT
STIMULANTS AND OTHER DRINKS

DO THIS NOW!

The Shopping List

Are the shops still open? There's no time like the present – write your basics list in your Notebook (use the back of it for lists) and head for the shops. Or if the shops are shut, make a list of what you're going to buy tomorrow.

Here are some suggestions for your basic store cupboard:

- Dried herbs and spices (e.g. mixed herbs – a good all rounder; chilli; paprika; tarragon – especially for chicken; rosemary – good with lamb; thyme and oregano.)

- Fresh herbs are even better if you're going to use them within a couple of days, or buy them in pots and they'll last a bit longer.

- Cooking oil (olive oil, sunflower, safflower or sesame)

- Cereals (steer clear of highly sweetened and processed cereals – even the plain bran ones have extra sugar. You can always add fresh or dried fruit for natural flavour and sweetening.)

- Dried Fruit

- Dried or tinned beans and lentils (e.g. chickpeas, kidney, haricot and mixed beans for salads.)

- Fresh garlic, chillies and ginger (these add flavour to lots of things and keep for quite a while in the fridge)

- Frozen vegetables and unsweetened fruit (for when you run out of fresh)

- Pasta

- Rice and other grains (e.g. bulgar wheat, couscous)

- Tins of tomatoes (for instant sauces)

- Tinned fish (e.g. tuna and sardines)

- Fresh fruit and vegetables to last a couple of days
- Nuts and seeds (almonds, brazils, hazelnuts, pumpkin seeds, sesame seeds, sunflower seeds, walnuts). These are good for adding to salads as well as for snacks.

Shopping Guidelines

You'll probably know some of these already, but here they are:

- Don't shop when you're hungry, and go when you're feeling awake and energetic rather than when you're tired.

- If you have children, try to avoid taking them with you!

- Take your list and stick to it if you can.

- Go for the simplest, purest foods, the less processed the better. Avoid added sugar, salt and chemicals (this includes artificial sweeteners).

- Wholefoods and unrefined grains have more nutritional value than refined and processed ones.

- Avoid slimming foods – they may have extra sugar and additives to compensate for being low in fat.

- Consider shopping online – then you won't be tempted to buy stuff you don't need.

Every household and every human being has different needs and habits, so you can adapt these suggestions to your own situation, but remember, Lighten Up is all about freeing you from food habits you want to break.

It doesn't matter if it doesn't work first time. After her first session on a recent Lighten Up course, Meena decided to re-think her kitchen. She went shopping first and when she came back with her bags of Foods To Focus On she couldn't find anywhere to put them. So she emptied the cupboards, ruthlessly tipping half-eaten packets of biscuits and slimming snacks into the bin – until she came to the bag of kettle chips. 'I can't bear to throw them out,' she thought. 'And I can't leave them there either.' The next minute she was sitting down in the middle of her half-unpacked shopping, finishing off the hand-fried salsa and mesquite crisps.

Later on in the book I'll be offering some ideas about what to do if your slimming programme runs into setbacks as Meena's did, but right now, you're running your own minesweeping exercise so that you can give yourself a head start. I want to make slimming simple for you right from the very beginning.

Lighten Up Lifestyle

So now you've sorted out your kitchen, what about the rest of your home? Does it reflect your current lifestyle, or the slimmer, fitter, healthier lifestyle you'd like to have?

I'm not suggesting you embark on a Feng Shui, clutter-clearing programme, but it's worth thinking about a couple of things:

- Could you limit eating to just one particular area? The kitchen? The dining room if you have one? If you decide to ban eating in bed or on the sofa, it's going to cut down the danger zones at home significantly.

- Is there somewhere where you have (or can make) the space to do a few simple exercises? Don't panic – I'm not leading up to an hour's aerobics every day – but it's useful to start thinking of your living space in terms of stretching and moving as well as resting.

First Steps Fitness

Remember the Fitness Pyramid in Chapter 1? Well now's the time to get started on the first level, which consists of four very simple exercises that introduce you to the importance of exercise and complement Fat Jar and Feel Good Fitness. You can split them up during the day, although we do suggest you try to do them together. See Chapter 6 for more details about home exercise.

1. Practising perfect posture

This exercise focuses you on holding your spine in total alignment, avoiding any unnecessary strain on your lower back. The position is commonly called Neutral Spine by fitness professionals. Doing this as often as you can, will help you to strengthen deep postural muscles in your lower back and stomach area, and it will also help you to stand taller and look slimmer!

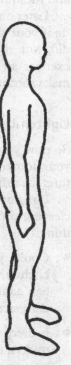

- Stand sideways in front of a mirror and arch your back as much as you can, sticking out your bottom and chest. Then go to the other extreme and round your shoulders and push your hips forward.

- Now that you've experienced and seen both extremes of posture, find a comfortable middle ground. You should be able to draw an imaginary line between your ear, shoulder, hip, knee and ankle.

- Keep your eyes straight ahead of you and imagine a golden thread is gently pulling you up from the crown of your head, elongating the back of your neck.

- With your hands on your waist, cough. Notice the muscles that work involuntarily when you cough. These are the muscles you want to recruit all the time – when standing, lying or sitting. Start by holding the Neutral Spine position for ten seconds. Repeat as often as you can. As you build up strength, you'll be able to hold them for longer until you automatically hold this posture all the time.

Once you can comfortably allocate these muscles, you can do this exercise any time and anywhere.

2. Squats

- Stand with your feet hip width apart, keeping your knees in line with your toes and your knees soft.

- Lower your bottom as if you're going to sit in a chair, bending your knees to a 90° angle. Keep your weight over your heels and your arms in front of you to counterbalance your body weight.

- Return to standing by pushing up through your heels.

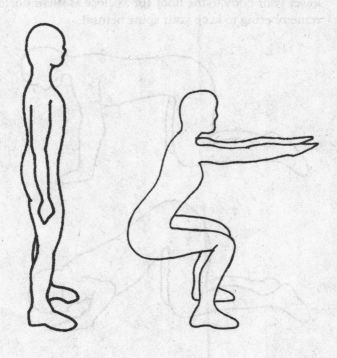

Throughout the movement, keep your spine neutral and ensure your knees are over your ankles.

You can begin this exercise by placing a secure chair behind you and lowering yourself to the point where you feel the chair under your bottom and then return to standing. This may make you feel safer until you become more comfortable with the movement.

Repeat 10–20 times.

3. Press Ups

- Kneel on your hands and knees, placing your hands directly under your shoulders and slightly wider than shoulder width apart. Keep your eyes to the floor, your spine neutral and your elbows soft. Bend your arms to lower your body to the floor (or as close as is comfortable), remembering to keep your spine neutral.

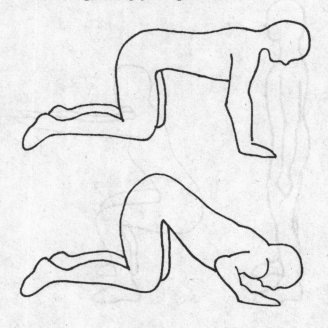

- Return to the starting position by pushing up through the palms of your hands.

- Repeat the movement 8–20 times. Rest and repeat sequence.

As you become stronger, change your body position by moving your knees further away from your hands, ensuring you keep your spine neutral.

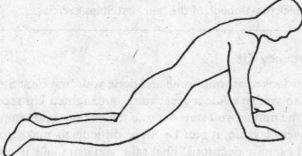

If you're just starting out, you may begin by performing a press up standing up against a wall. Your arms, head and tummy all keep the same position as before.

4. Arm Curl

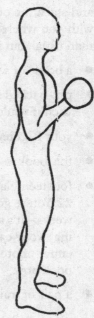

- Stand or sit with a neutral spine. If standing, make sure your knees aren't locked.

- Hold a dumb-bell (or a soup tin, or whatever is convenient) in each hand with your palms facing forward, then curl your arms up alternately keeping your elbows in tight at your waist.

- Keep the rest of your body still.

Use a weight that feels tough after 12–15 repetitions.
You can also do this exercise with any object of a decent
weight, e.g. bags of shopping, bottles of water (you can vary
the amount of water in the bottles according to your strength),
boxes of washing powder.

(DO THIS NOW!)

Have a quick run-through of the four First Steps exercises.

The Emergency Kit

You've now looked at your home and done your first First Steps
exercises, so you've made a great start, but Lighten Up recog-
nises that the minute you step out into the stresses and tempta-
tions of everyday life, it can be more difficult to make good
eating and exercise decisions. That said, you can make it easier
and stack the odds in your favour by taking an Emergency Kit
with you wherever you go. This may mean taking a bigger bag
than usual, but it's a good habit to get into, so collect up:

- a bottle of water

- pre-packed snacks (fruit, nuts, raisins – maybe even a sandwich if you're going to be out for long)

- your Lighten Up Notebook and a pen

- this book

- fourteen blank copies of the Food Profile, as shown in page
  22. You're going to be filling it out every day for the first two
  weeks – it's a brilliant way of revealing (and therefore changing) your eating habits – but it will be much simpler if you
  either photocopy or draw each day's Profile into your Notebook now.

- a pair of trainers

Now you're ready – but you aren't going to start just yet. You still have one more important area to clear and prepare. There's no point in setting up a motivating environment if you still haven't cleared the mental space you're going to need for the new slimming ideas I'll be introducing.

Slimming Myths

We'll begin by clearing out some of the old myths that may still be taking up valuable mind space.

DO THIS NOW!

How Many of These Myths Do You Subscribe To?	Yes	No
1 I've got fat genes		
2 I'm too busy to exercise		
3 Dieting is the only way to lose weight		
4 Everybody puts on weight as they get older		
5 The only way to lose weight is to cut out fat		
6 Breakfast is the most important meal of the day		
7 I can't lose weight because my lifestyle involves a lot of socialising/driving/travelling/sitting down		
8 I have a family to feed so eating healthy food is not an option for me		
9 I'll always have to watch my weight – it's not natural for me to be slim		

The Truth About the Myths

1. Specific medical conditions aside, there is a slight tendency for some people to accumulate more fat cells than others but the difference is very small and everybody can be slim if they eat healthy food and take enough exercise. Families who share weight problems are more likely to be out of shape because of shared eating and exercise patterns than because they share genes.

2. Taking time out to be more active helps you use your time more efficiently for the rest of the day. Human beings were designed for movement and if you spend most of your time lying and sitting down your mental and physical efficiency is likely to be impaired. Activity is an energiser and exercise improves your quality of sleep as well as your mood and concentration.

3. Drastic dieting may put you at risk of not getting the full range of nutrients you need, and tends to make you think more about food than you normally would. When you stop dieting you will probably regain the weight very quickly.

4. A lot of people gain weight as they get older primarily because they tend to become less active and lose some of their fat-burning muscle mass year by year. But you don't have to, and the older you get, the more important it is to stay active. There are plenty of role models out there: Honor Blackman, Harrison Ford, Susan Sarandon, Sting, Sigourney Weaver, Clint Eastwood and Lulu, to name just a few.

5. Cutting out fat completely is a bad idea because your body needs a certain amount of it to function. Some fats are better for you than others so take a look at Chapter 7 and check which are which.

6. Yes, breakfast is important because it gets your metabolism going in the morning. However, it doesn't necessarily mean eating as soon as you wake up. So if you don't feel hungry before you leave home in the morning, take a banana or a sandwich with you so that you're ready as soon as your stomach starts asking for food.

7. You can always find reasons not to eat well or exercise regularly, but there are plenty of people who socialise, drive, travel and sit down a lot who maintain good activity levels and balanced eating patterns. It's possible – and the payoff is your health.

8. The best thing you can do for your family is set them a good example by providing plenty of healthy food. Your children may need more calories than you, and very active teenagers may need to eat a lot more than their parents. It's a good idea to offer them plenty of fruit, salad and vegetables as well as all the other Foods To Focus On, and suggest that everybody eats when they are hungry and stops when they are full.

9. For most people, it's natural to be slim, fit and healthy. It's just a question of fitting your lifestyle to your expectations.

DO THIS NOW!

The Commitment

Open your Lighten Up Notebook and write your Commitment on the first page:

The Motivation Scale:

Low									High
1	2	3	4	5	6	7	8	9	10

On a scale of one to ten my current motivation level is ......

I have checked off and put aside all my personal slimming myths.

I have decided to complete the course and try out all the Lighten Up techniques over the next four weeks. I owe it to myself to give myself the best possible chance of success.

Signed...

Date...

Chapter 3

The Lighten Up Four-Week Weight Loss Plan

Week One

WEEK ONE STARTER

FIRST:

- *Re-read the Commitment you wrote in your Notebook (or on page 34 of Chapter 2) and check your motivation level again. Has it changed?*

Tomorrow you'll be starting the four-week programme and now's the time to decide how you're going to read the book.

Ideally, you'll be reading this Starter section and having a quick look through Day One now. Then, starting tomorrow, set aside just ten or fifteen minutes every morning to read the day's section thoroughly.

On the other hand, if you're not a morning person or you're pressed for time in the mornings, you can read this Starter section and skim through all of Week One right now. Then you'll need just five minutes each morning to check what you'll be doing.

What will work best for you?

The Lighten Up Three-Part Programme

Every day we'll be giving you three pieces of the Lighten Up jigsaw: a motivational piece, an eating piece and a piece about exercise. Over the next four weeks the pieces will fit together and the ones that are going to become part of your long-term lifestyle will be permanently fixed.

Of course, not everything works for everybody, but day by day, and week by week, you'll become aware of what works for you.

Lose Those Scales

We'll be talking about habits and how you can control them later in the book, but weighing yourself is a poor slimming habit you can get rid of right away, because your weight fluctuates for lots of reasons other than fat.

This is what weighing-in daily has done for you:

- maintained your obsession with your weight

- supported your belief that losing weight is difficult

- made you miserable

Chances are, the one thing it hasn't done is motivate you.

But how will you measure your progress without any scales? If that thought makes you even more anxious than your daily weigh-ins, you can make one last check. On the Lighten Up courses we hand out measurement sheets for those who want to use them. They aren't really necessary but they make people feel better. You will see and feel the difference in your size and shape over a few weeks anyway, but for now, if it gives you more confidence, go ahead and take your measurements. You can fill the table in right here on the page, but it's best to photocopy it or just write it all down on a blank piece of paper and put it away out of sight until you've finished the programme.

(To get the most accurate result, make sure you're wearing the same clothes and being measured by the same person, if not yourself.)

Measurements	Pre-programme	After the programme
Chest: (measure at the widest point, i.e. on the nipple line)		
Upper non-dominant arm: (measure halfway between your shoulder and elbow)		
Waist:		
Hips: (measure at widest point)		
Upper Leg – specify left or right: (measure halfway between the top of your leg and your knee)		
Calf – specify left or right: (measure the widest point)		
Weight:		
Clothing Size:		

Checklist

1. Make sure you've got your Emergency Kit from Chapter 2 – remember?

    - Bottle of water
    - Pre-packed snacks
    - Notebook & pen
    - This book
    - Blank copies of the Food Profile
    - A pair of trainers

2. Did you do the mental and physical space clearing exercise? Even if you only made a few changes, it's a start. Is there anything else you want to do before you go for Day One?

DAY ONE

FIRST: _____

Remember it's a good idea to keep this book as well as your Notebook and pen with you as you go through the four weeks. You'll be noticing patterns and habits and changes you want to make – as well as all the positive changes you've already made – and you'll probably want to write them down.

Today's challenges . . .

Motivation

Defining your goals

Using the Feel Good Scale

Eating

Identifying your danger areas

Using the Hunger Scale

Exercise

Remembering to do your First Steps session

The Sedentary Circle

Motivation

We're going to start with something incredibly easy, but absolutely essential. It's almost impossible to stick with anything – whether it's giving up smoking, losing weight or studying for exams – unless you have a really clear idea of why you want to do it, and what difference it will make to your life. So, the first thing you need to do is define your goals right now.

Challenge: Defining your goals

What is your personal goal for this course? You may find that you have more than one so just jot down whatever you can think of: what you want to achieve, how you want to feel and how you might change what you do.

_____

_____

_____

_____

Make sure all your intentions are positive. Say what you want ('I want to be slimmer') not what you don't want ('I want to stop feeling fat').

Now that you've defined where you want to get to, let's pause for a moment and look at where you are right now.

In Chapter 2 I asked you to check where you were on a Motivation Scale of one to ten, and I'll be asking you to do that regularly over the next four weeks. If you notice a rise or a dip in your motivation, check what caused it. You might notice that certain foods give you energy while others send you to sleep, or that getting out in the sunshine makes you cheerful, and staying indoors makes you feel fed up. You'll only learn these things if you get into the habit of checking how you feel instead of just reaching for quick fixes when it all gets too much.

So here's a variation on the Motivation Scale: it's called the Feel Good Scale and it's very important because the more positive you feel about yourself – and the better you treat yourself - the easier it will be for you to achieve your goals.

Challenge: Using the Feel Good Scale

On a scale of one to ten, right now, how do you feel about yourself?

Hopeless			Could Be Better				Very Positive		
1	2	3	4	5	6	7	8	9	10

There are a lot of scales in Lighten Up (other than weighing ones of course) because it's important to be aware of how you're feeling as you make progress on the course.

Putting numbers on feelings may seem strange at first, but it will help you measure your feelings about food. As the saying goes, 'if you can measure it, you can manage it', and putting a figure on something somehow makes it seem more predictable and easier to control.

Eating

Your Personal Eating Plan

We're moving on now to the Eating part of the programme for today and I'll be introducing you to two really important Lighten Up techniques. The first is using the Food Profile to help you identify the kinds of food that give you the hardest time.

You'll have noticed by now that I haven't given you lists of foods you should and shouldn't eat. Instead, the Lighten Up programme provides an easy formula for working out what you need – which is a lot better than dictating what you're allowed.

Do you remember filling in the two Food Profile circles in Chapter 2? Well, go back and have another look at where you put your crosses. What do you see? What's the balance between Foods To Limit and Foods To Focus On? Assuming that what's in your kitchen bears some relationship to what goes into you, chances are you're looking at a reasonably accurate picture of your current eating habits. And while it's possible that you simply tend to eat too much of everything, most people have quite specific weaknesses.

So what do your Food Profiles tell you about your weak spots? Looking at the two circles, where do you see your danger zones? Sweet things like chocolates and biscuits? Savoury snacks like crisps? Working out what it is that's likely to trip you up is a crucial step towards successful slimming, so make a list

---

Challenge: My danger areas are:

1. _____

2. _____

3. _____

Just for today, avoid them all.

here of your three toughest potential eating hazards. And if they tempt you today, eat something healthier instead.

The Hunger Scale

The second healthy eating technique you need for Day One is the Hunger Scale. One of the main problems with slimming is that so many of us eat for so many reasons other than hunger. And if you eat when you aren't hungry, your body will store what you don't need for later.

The Hunger Scale is an essential tool which you'll be using for the rest of your life.

Not hungry						Fairly hungry		Danger Zone Starving	
1	2	3	4	5	6	7	8	9	10

This basic diagram is all you need to think about every time you sit down to eat. It's very simple, and it's designed to fix the 'how much?' and 'how often?' questions that diets don't give you good answers for. The real answer to both questions is the same: *Eat when you're hungry and stop when you're full.*

Challenge: Using the Hunger Scale

When are you next planning to eat? Before you decide to put something in your mouth, stop, and ask yourself how hungry you are on a scale of one to ten. If you're less than six or seven, you aren't hungry enough to eat. Even if your watch tells you it's time for a meal, have a drink of water or do a First Steps session instead.

From now on you'll be checking your personal Hunger Scale every time you think about food. If you don't know exactly where you are on the scale, just pretend you do. It will be close enough.

Exercise

Last, but definitely not least, let's take a look at the third part of the programme for today – exercise.

First Steps

You've already started to build up your Fat Burning Pyramid with First Steps Fitness, and that's your first and most important exercise goal for today:

Challenge: Remember to do your First Steps session

If possible, choose the time of day when you're usually least active – that way you'll get the most benefit from them.

The Exercise Wheel

Tomorrow I'll be introducing you to Fat Jar Fitness which is the next level on the pyramid, but, first, let's run a check on your current level of activity.

This could be called the Sedentary Circle because when most people fill it in for the first time they are shocked at how low their activity levels are. Each of the segments in the examples below represents one hour of the day. I've filled in a couple to give you examples of a typical working day and a typical weekend day.

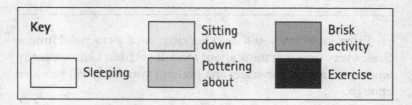

Working day

  6 hours sleep
12 hours sitting (2 hours car, 6 hours
     sitting in office,
     4 hours TV)
  3 hours pottering at
     home and work
  2 hours brisk walking
     dog and brisk
     walking in lunch-
     break
  1 hour exercise at
     gym

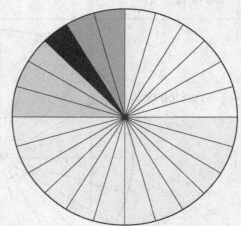

Weekend day

  8 hours sleep
  7 hours sitting (1 hour car, 2 hours
     cinema, 1 hour TV,
     2 hours dinner/lunch/pub)
  5 hours pottering around
     house and in shops
  4 hours brisk walking
     dog, cycling with
     kids, gardening

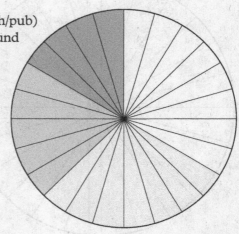

Challenge: Using the Exercise Wheel

Shade in the empty wheels according to your own lifestyle –
and be honest!

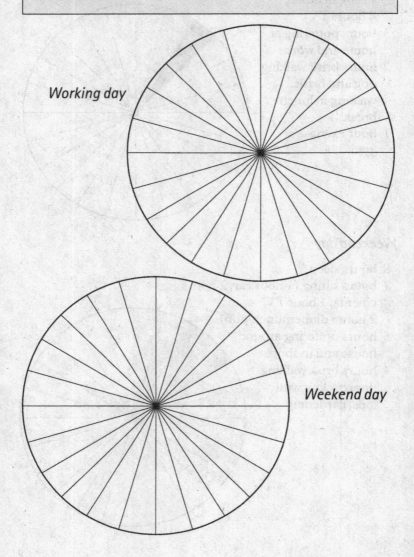

Working day

Weekend day

The categories are:

Sleeping

Sitting down	this includes driving, sitting on a train or bus, desk work and watching TV
Pottering about	light housework, shopping, office and shop work
Brisk activity	walking, cycling, gardening, vacuuming, scrubbing floors
Exercise	running, lifting weights, playing tennis, swimming etc.

How much of your day involves parking your body while your brain gets on with life? In spite of the clear link between low levels of activity and high levels of obesity, most of us still move around as little as possible. So it's time to think about being more active.

Of course, our lifestyle is against us. In 1951 only 14% of the population owned a car, but by 2000 73% of us had our own wheels.*

In 1955, television was only broadcast for five hours a day to the 30% of households who actually owned a set. Multiple channels are now broadcast twenty-four hours a day and the average viewer watches more than twenty-four hours of TV in a week. Which leaves only six days out of the seven for work, sleep and more active forms of recreation.

Does it matter?

Yes, it does matter. Our bodies were designed for movement – and even our brains work more efficiently if we carry them around in a healthy body. Yet most of us spend more hours sitting down than anything else.

*Department of Transport, 2002.

DO THIS NOW!

When you shaded in your circle, did you see plenty of potential exercise space? Or are you tired and stressed enough with life as it is? How we spend our time tends to reflect our values in life, so take a minute to think about what priority you would put on the following activities in your life. I've listed them here in alphabetical order and you can put them in number order below. You can add in any special priorities of your own.

Commitments to family and other people

Health and fitness (taking care of myself)

Relaxation

Work

1 _____

2 _____

3 _____

4 _____

What does this tell you? It's not as straightforward as it might appear to be – here are a couple of clues:

- If you neglect your health, ultimately you will become a liability rather than an asset to the people you care for.

- Exercise can be both physically energising and mentally relaxing.

You'll have noticed that Day One of your four-week plan seems to have been largely about checking up on where you are. Why is that important? Wouldn't it be better if I just got on with the programme and told you what to do?

The answer, of course, is no. The reason that so many people try and fail to lose weight is that they don't put in the time up front to make sure they are ready to succeed. You may have started loads of diets in the past feeling fully prepared to suffer, but you probably weren't prepared to succeed.

You wouldn't climb a mountain or run a marathon or sit an exam without preparing for it first, would you? Well, slimming's the same. Ask yourself:

- Am I motivated enough?
- Have I set myself at least one clear, positive goal?
- How positive am I feeling?

DAY TWO

FIRST: _____

*Take a look at how you're getting on with your Notebook. If you use it
often enough, it will give you support and help you become more
aware of what you're doing and what you want to change. After all,
you can't change something you don't know about, can you?*

Today's Challenges . . .

Motivation

Using the Hunger Scale to identify your eating triggers

Eating

Using the Food Profile

Exercise

Getting started with Fat Jar Fitness

Designing your ideal Exercise Wheel

Motivation

You've had a day to get used to using the Hunger Scale, and now it's time to start using it to analyse what – other than hunger – is driving your eating habits. So:

Challenge: Using the Hunger Scale to identify your eating triggers

In your Notebook, write down where you are on the Hunger Scale every time you eat today. If you are below six or seven, write down what triggered you to eat *other than hunger*. Were you bored? Were you feeling stressed and that sugar rush made you feel better? Were you tired? Was it just that the people around you were eating? Be honest.

Eating

Food Profile

It's time to look at the Food Profile in more detail. If you're not sure about anything, check the Food Lists in Chapter 7.

How does it work?

You already used the Food Profile in Chapter 2 when you cleared out your kitchen cupboards, and for the next week you'll be using it to keep a record of everything you eat and drink.

This isn't about controlling what you eat, or beating yourself up about it, it's just a very graphic, quick and simple way to get a picture of your eating habits as they start to change.

Start at the centre of the Food Profile and work out towards the edge. Every time you have something to eat or drink, put a cross on a line, in the appropriate section. If you run out of lines (for example you might drink a lot of water on a particular day) just put your crosses outside the circle.

Don't try to be too precise – the Food Profile is rough and ready. Some foods fall into more than one category, some meals have lots of ingredients and it's hard to separate them out. Just give it your best guess and by the end of the week it will give you a pretty accurate picture of your eating habits.

Challenge: Using the Food Profile

Draw or photocopy six Food Profiles into your Notebook – one for each day left this week. Then fill it in throughout the day. Remember to include what you drink as well as what you eat.

Foods To Focus On

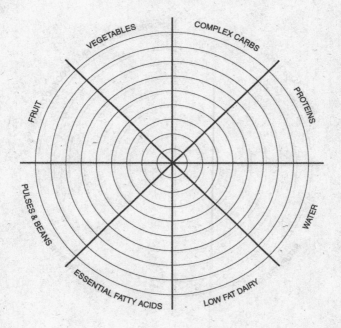

Fruit
Vegetables

Complex Carbohydrates (bread, cereals, grains, potatoes)
Proteins (lean meat, fish, poultry)

Pulses, Lentils and Beans
Essential Fatty Acids (oily fish, sunflower oil, olive oil)
Low Fat Dairy
Water

Remember: it's a good idea to drink around two litres of water a day and eat at least the Department of Health minimum recommendation of five servings of fruit and vegetables.

Foods To Limit

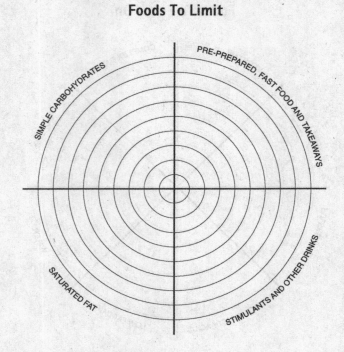

Simple Carbohydrates (sugar)
Pre-prepared food, fast food and takeaways
Saturated fat (full fat dairy)

Stimulants (tea, coffee, alcohol, chocolate)

Remember: if you're eating enough of the Foods To Focus On, then you can survive without any of these – although we don't expect you to cut them out completely. But if this circle is full while Foods To Focus On is empty, it means you're putting a strain on your body, depriving it of some of the nutrients it needs, and lowering your chances of becoming – and staying - slim and healthy.

Exercise

Remember the Fat Burning Pyramid on page 17? You've already incorporated First Steps Fitness into your daily routine – and you'll want to keep going with these exercises – but it's also time to move on to the next level.

Fat Jar Fitness

Next week I'll introduce you to the Lighten Up approach to Feel Good Fitness and suggest some ways you could start having more fun, but first, we'll take a look at what we call Fat Jar Fitness and see what you can do to turn your body into a fat burning machine without giving it too much of a shock.

Get yourself a glass jar and put it somewhere conspicuous – somewhere you'll see it several times a day. We're going to call this glass jar your Fat Jar, and it's a visual aid to help you keep track of how much more active you can be on a daily basis. Put ten to fifteen pence in it every time you take ten to fifteen minutes of continuous brisk exercise such as walking, cycling, gardening or housework. These are what we call Fat Burning Pills and once you've got a jar full of them you can reward yourself with a book or CD you've always wanted, or a trip to the cinema.

Challenge: Getting started with Fat Jar Fitness

Today take two Fat Burning Pills (five, ten or fifteen pence, depending on how many minutes), but remember that what constitutes a Fat Burning Pill is, up to a point, defined by how active you already are:

- If you're totally inactive at present, for whatever reason, simply tailor the two Fat Burning Pills to what you can do. Even if it's just walking for five minutes instead of

---

the fifteen I've suggested, the important thing is that you're honest with yourself and you do it.

- If you're already pretty active, add in two brisk fifteen-minute Fat Burning Pills, preferably at a time when you're normally inactive. If you sit at a desk in an office all day, for example, try going out at lunchtime and walking fast for fifteen minutes. When you leave work perhaps you could walk for fifteen minutes before catching the bus a bit closer to home. These Fat Burning Pills really don't have to interfere with your existing lifestyle.

If time is a problem, then you can either:

- Take two ten-minute breaks instead, or

- Split the two fifteen-minute chunks up into six separate five-minute breaks. (Again, if you work in an office, walk down to the ground floor and then walk up as many flights of stairs as you can. Everybody will think you're very busy rather than taking a quick break, and you'll find that as your body speeds up so will your mind, making you more efficient when you return to your desk.)

However active you already are, it's very important that you do this. It may not be physically very challenging, but you're starting to test the limits and patterns you've currently set yourself so that you can see what can be challenged or changed.

Fat Jar Benefits

This sort of exercise is fantastically good for you because:

- Enjoyable, comfortable activity is the best way to burn fat.

- You can be more active without moving far from your comfort zone.

- In fact, most people on Lighten Up courses surprise themselves by starting to enjoy a more active lifestyle.

Love it or leave it

Our exercise advice is based on a single principle – the pleasure principle. If you don't enjoy it, we don't want you to do it. So choose a form of exercise that you'll enjoy, whatever it is, and you'll be surprised at the results.

Maybe right now you can't really imagine what it would be like to enjoy exercising regularly, but I'm often amazed at just how quickly some of the most dedicated career couch potatoes can learn to flick the pleasure switch when it comes to exercise.

Exercise Wish Wheel

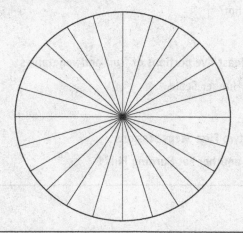

Challenge: Designing your ideal Exercise Wheel

This time, don't fill in what you actually do, or don't do. Shade it in according to what you'd *like* to be doing by the end of the course. You can then refer back to it later and see if you're getting closer to your ideal exercise programme.

DAY THREE

FIRST:

Identify any belief you may have about yourself that might be getting in the way of you being slim. Could you let go of that belief – just for the next few weeks?

Today's Challenges . . .

Motivation

Thinking slim?

Eating

Eating at least five portions of fruit and vegetables

Using the Hunger Scale

Exercise

Fitting in two First Steps sessions

Adding in another Fat Burning Pill

Motivation

Body Image

So many people come to Lighten Up and tell me they feel like failures. Over and over again, they've tried to lose weight and failed. They've lost it and gained it and lost it and gained it all over again.

'The times I've been slim,' said Victoria, 'I never felt like it was really me. Deep down I know that I'm a big woman, like my Mum. Occasionally, I lose some weight for a special occasion – like I'm losing it now for my daughter's wedding – but I'm just acting slim and I'll go back to being me when it's all over. To be honest, it's quite a relief when I've been through one of my thin phases and then I go back to not worrying about it any more.'

'Has it ever occurred to you,' I asked her, 'to give yourself credit for all the effort you've put into being overweight?'

She looked at me as if I was mad.

'Being overweight is normal, it's being slim that's hard,' she said. 'I can't think of a single one of my friends who is totally happy with the way they are.'

Many of us tend to choose friends who think like we do and share our problems. Imagine how you'd feel if most of your friends *didn't* worry about their weight – if you were the odd one out? Of course, friends like that may be hard to find because more and more men and women are becoming obsessed about their size. Various recent surveys have all produced similarly depressing statistics:

- only 25% of young women are happy with their weight *

- 99% of women are dissatisfied with their bodies †

- only one in ten British women is happy with her body ‡

* The Bread for Life Campaign, 'Pressure to be Perfect' report, 1998.
† *New Woman* Body Survey, 2001.
‡ Schools Health Education Unit, October 2000.

You may not be happy with the shape you're in right now, but you probably put more effort than you think into getting there. If you don't believe me, check this.

DO THIS NOW!

	Yes	No
● Have I spent time in the past thinking about what I was allowed to eat?		
● Have I spent time thinking about what I wasn't allowed to eat?		
● Have I spent more time thinking about food than eating it?		
● Have I counted calories?		
● Have I weighed portions?		
● Have I thought about social events in terms of what I could and couldn't eat?		
● Have I ever skipped a social event because I wasn't sure I could cope?		
● Have I taken up exercise I hated in the hope of losing weight?		
● Have I ever spent more time beating myself up over eating a chocolate bar than actually eating it?		
● Do I usually know what I weigh?		

Even if you didn't answer yes to all of those questions, you probably scored pretty high – most people do – and that means you've put a lot of effort and energy into being the fat person you think you are. So accept your Oscar – you've put in a great performance.

But now it's time to move on.

Challenge: Thinking Slim

Think about the alternative to being the shape you are now. How different would things be if you were slim? Either in your Notebook or below, list three things you would do differently if you were already slim.

1. _____

2. _____

3. _____

Eating

Food Profile

How did you get on with the Food Profile yesterday? You'll be continuing to use it for the next few weeks. Just put in the crosses every time you eat, and by the end of this week you'll already be able to see the patterns, changes and gaps.

Foods To Focus On and Foods To Limit

Although the average person eats fewer calories than fifty years ago, a much larger proportion of the population is overweight. Our diet has changed pretty drastically in fifty years and now includes far more sugar and fat than our bodies need.

The huge rise in pre-prepared meals, takeaways and fast food are partly to blame and, if you've been wondering why these are Foods To Limit, here's the reason: they are generally relatively high in sugar, fat and additives and low in nutritional value. Even foods which are labelled 'low fat' and 'good for you' are often misleading.

The key to healthy eating is to go for food that doesn't have a label. Anything with a long list of unfamiliar ingredients is a second-best option, and some of the best, healthiest and tastiest forms of unlabelled foods are so obvious that they're easy to forget. They are of course fruit and vegetables.

As you probably know, we're all advised to eat at least five portions of fruit and vegetables every day, although apparently very few of us do - in spite of the fact that they're fantastically good for us.

If you think you don't like fruit or vegetables you may not have tried enough different varieties – or perhaps you've eaten them under-ripe or over-ripe or badly cooked. Give them another go. Don't eat anything you really don't like, but there are always options: if you don't like broccoli for dinner, have a banana for breakfast instead. And taste as wide a range of exotic fruit as you can – if you're bored with apples and oranges, go for something more exotic like mangoes, kiwis, nectarines and figs.

Challenge: Using the Food Profile

Make sure you put at least five crosses in Fruit and Vegetables today

---

Challenge: Using the Hunger Scale

Are you using the Hunger Scale every time you think about food? What are you doing when you don't register high enough to eat? Your body may be suggesting food simply because you've been sitting down too long or allowing yourself to get thirsty. Before you jump to conclusions about needing food, try a few alternative options first. For example:

- drink a couple of glasses of water – you might just be thirsty;

- move around a bit – go for a walk round the block or the office. You might just be bored or tired;

- try a First Steps session or take a Fat Burning Pill – you might just be low on energy and a few exercises will perk you up.

Exercise

Lastly, let's take a look at how you're getting on with building your Fat Burning Pyramid, starting with the baseline – your First Steps Fitness. Are they becoming part of your daily routine yet?

Challenge: Fitting in two First Steps sessions

If you're worried about whether you have time, here are some ideas. Do the exercises:

- While you're running a bath.

- As soon as you get home from work – at that danger point where habit tells you to head for the fridge.

- In the time it takes pasta to cook.

- Just before bed.

Fat Jar Fitness

And how about Fat Jar Fitness? Are there any Fat Burning Pills in your jar? Remember, those pills can be any size you want and although we recommend fifteen minutes, the dose really depends on you.

You can vary either the time or the intensity – or both – just as long as you make an effort to do *something*. If you aren't well, if you've been inactive for a long time or if your ability to move is limited for any reason, just do what you can.

Challenge: Adding in another Fat Burning Pill

That's a total of three Fat Jar Fitness sessions today. If you're not sure you've got time, how about doing fifteen minutes of gentle step or body toning exercises while you watch your favourite soap? Or have a look at your Exercise Wheel and find a place where you have more than an hour of sitting down, and fit in a session there.

While you're doing your Fat Jar Fitness today, ask yourself a few key questions. Are you noticing:

- increased or decreased energy ?

- increased or decreased appetite?

- increased or decreased concentration?

- a change of mood?

It may be too soon for you to notice any real changes, but when you do, write them in your Notebook.

DAY FOUR

FIRST: _____

Think back over yesterday – what was the most useful technique or piece of information for you? Have you used it yet?

Today's Challenges . . .

Motivation

Finding your Personal Plus Factor

Eating

Identifying an eating habit you'd like to change

Checking the Food Profile

Exercise

Turning an everyday task into a Fat Burning Pill

Timing your Fat Burning Pills

Motivation

Being Your Own Role Model

You've accepted your Oscar, and you've recognised all the skill, determination and effort you've put into getting the result you didn't want. All those years of dieting, being obsessive about your weight, ignoring the messages your body sent you and firmly believing you were destined to be fat are behind you now. You're ready to play a new role.

But remember all the positive things you did as well.

(DO THIS NOW!)

Being your own Role Model

Think of the times you made a decision and went right ahead and did it, regardless of obstacles. It doesn't matter whether it turned out to be right or wrong. It's the process that matters. For example:

You bought a car

You moved to a place of your own

You changed jobs

You went to college

You passed some exams

You gave up work to look after the kids

You learned to dance

You got married

You became independent

You adopted a cat

You started a business

You saved up for a holiday

You won an award for something

What was it for you?

_____

_____

_____

Once you've chosen a memory or two, run through them in your mind. Enjoy them for a few seconds and then, while they're still with you, make a firm commitment to yourself to be slimmer. Leave yourself no other option. True commitment to a decision unlocks the energy to achieve it. While you're thinking about commitments, flip back to page 34 in Chapter 2, re-read what you wrote and, if you think it will help you, write it out again.

Challenge: Finding your Personal Plus Factor

Think about what you've got going for you that will help you stick with this four-week course. It could be:

● Something about you: a personal attribute perhaps, like determination.

● A Lighten Up technique: you've already started using the Hunger Scale and introduced a regular First Step session and brisk exercise into your everyday life. These two factors alone could make a permanent, positive difference to the way you look and the way you feel.

● An external factor in your life: sometimes it's a doctor's warning or a relationship under threat, or sometimes it's something positive, like a new job that makes us want to upgrade our appearance.

Whatever your Personal Plus Factor is, you can make it work for you. Write it down in your Notebook and post it on your fridge as well.

Eating

You and your habits

Everyone's eating habits are different – we've all got our own particular weaknesses. However, you can't eliminate the habits you want to leave behind unless you first work out what they are. You started doing this on Day Two when you analysed why you ate without being hungry, but now you're going to take it a step further and look at *what* you eat instead of *why*.

Challenge: Identifying an eating habit you'd like to change

What's your problem area? It could be doughnuts at work, popcorn when you watch TV, biscuits when you get home, late night ice creams or fried breakfasts when you travel. Or perhaps it's going back for seconds when you know you're full, finishing the children's meal before you have dinner or grabbing snacks when you're shopping. Whatever it is, write it down in your Notebook.

Now write two or three ideas of ways to fix that habit . For example:

- Dipping into your Emergency Kit.

- Waiting until you're really, truly hitting the Hunger Scale at six or higher and then picking something from Foods To Focus On.

- Distracting yourself with First Steps or some Fat Jar Fitness.

Survival Shopping

It's much easier to clean up your eating habits if you've always got something healthy to hand, so have a look back at the basic store cupboard list in Chapter 2. You've now spent a few days filling in the Food Profile, so you've probably got some new ideas of your own to include as well. If you're feeling stuck, check the recipe ideas at the back of this book.

The Food Profile

The contents of your kitchen may be looking more like Foods To Focus On now, but what have you actually been eating? Open your Notebook and look back at your Food Profiles. Are there any totally blank sections in Foods To Focus On over the past couple of days? The ones most people miss out on are pulses, lentils and beans and the essential fatty acids – and if you're curious about why you need them, take a look at Chapter 7.

Challenge: Checking the Food Profile

In your Notebook write down two things that you don't usually eat from Foods To Focus On and make sure you do eat them today. If you hardly ever have pulses, for example, look at the recipes in Chapter 8, or make your own low-fat hummus (page 301).

Exercise

What you do is just as important as what you eat if you want to be slim. Our bodies were designed for movement, and the key to success is incorporating more of it into everyday life. However, there's a lot of popular nonsense around about exercise, so we'll clear up a few misconceptions right now.

Exercise Myths and Truths

Myth	Truth
If I exercise I'll end up looking like Arnold Schwarzenegger.	Exercise builds muscle which burns fat, weighs more than fat and takes up less space – but you won't look like Arnie unless you want to (and even then, it's very unlikely).
Exercise is painful and boring, just thinking about it makes me depressed.	Exercise releases 'happy' chemicals which improve your mood.
Exercise will wear me out – I won't have any energy for anything else.	Exercise energises you – a reasonable amount of exercise will make you energetic. it's inertia that makes you sluggish.
If I exercise, I'll just want to eat more.	Exercise helps you regulate your appetite.★

★ According to research carried out by scientists at the US Department of Energy's Brookhaven National Laboratory in New York in 2001, exercise increases the number of dopamine receptors in the brain. Tests showed that obese people's brain cells contained relatively few dopamine receptors, and the fatter they were, the fewer they had. Dopamine is a neurotransmitter (a substance that helps messages pass between brain cells) that seems to regulate the desire to eat – but if brain cells have few dopamine receptors, dopamine can't work.

So, when you think of exercising, think of the feeling you'll have afterwards and don't waste time on exercise you don't enjoy. One of your challenges today is to make it part of your daily life, rather than a chore.

Challenge: Turning an everyday task into a Fat Burning Pill

Think of an everyday task that could also be a Fat Burning Pill, for example:

- going to the shops
- walking the dog
- taking the children to school or going to work

Challenge: Timing your Fat Burning Pills

Are your three Fat Burning Pills spread fairly evenly throughout the day? If not, and if your daily schedule makes it at all possible, see if you can space them out a little more.

DAY FIVE

FIRST:

Have a quick look at your Notebook for the past four days and see if you notice anything you didn't realise before – it could be about eating, exercise, motivation, or all three.

Today's Challenges . . .

Motivation

Naming and shaming your Duck

Eating

Pacing yourself

The Hunger Scale Danger Zone

Exercise

Taking a fourth Fat Burning Pill

First Steps Fitness

Motivation

Over the years I've been working with Lighten Up, three questions have come up time and time again:

- Why is slimming so difficult?

- Why does it always go wrong – even when I start a diet that seems to be going well at first?

- Why can't I feel in control of my body and my eating habits?

The answer to all three questions is the same: dieting won't help you stay slim because it's about living by somebody else's (often arbitrary) set of rules. Successful slimming is about *you* and *your* body. It's totally personal. It's about getting to know yourself better instead of fighting a constant battle about what you should and shouldn't eat.

As you've probably noticed, a lot of Lighten Up is about awareness. Until you know exactly what you're doing and why you're doing it, you can't start to change it.

Meet the Duck

Lighten Up owes a lot to sports psychology – the science of using your mind to help your body. Athletes and slimmers both tend to sabotage themselves without realising it when they constantly talk to themselves about failure. Whether it's missed shots or missed target weights, the focus tends to be on what's going wrong rather than what's going right.

Over the years at Lighten Up we've started calling that internal pessimist the Duck – simply because somebody's voice, way back when, happened to sound like Donald Duck. We all carry one around with us and, whatever yours sounds like, you might find it helps to give it a name and tell it to shut up.

Challenge: Naming and shaming your Duck

Over the next couple of days, take the time to listen to the way you talk to yourself. What is that voice in your head saying to you about being slim? Is it encouraging you? Or telling you how difficult it's going to be? What (or who) does it sound like? Once you've accepted that it's there and faced up to it, you can start to argue back, forcefully, until it gets too weak to torment you any more.

Eating

Quick and Easy

A lot of Lighten Up techniques are very quick and simple, and this is one of the most effective. One of the most frequent reasons for eating too much is also one of the easiest to fix, and you probably know what it is already – it's eating too fast.

Unlike lions and tigers, we aren't designed to eat a lot all in one go and then survive for days until the next kill. Regardless of what the food looks like – or the amount everyone else is eating – your gut feeling is your best guide to how much you need to eat, but once you feel bloated it's too late. So, you need to slow down in order to listen to your body.

Challenge: Pacing yourself

Slow down. Taste your food and chew it slowly. Most importantly, listen to your stomach when it tells you you're full. If you think you've reached that point, remove yourself from temptation. Take your plate to the kitchen, leave the table or, if you're in a restaurant, put your knife and fork together and sit back in your chair. It won't work every time, but those physical movements are a strong sign to yourself and everybody else that you've finished, and that can be a psychological deterrent.

If you think you might be full but you're not sure, you probably are. Just wait twenty minutes – preferably away from the food. If that's not possible, focus on something else, like talking to your fellow diners. When your twenty minutes is up you can ask yourself again and, if you're still hungry, have a bit more.

Eating triggers

For the last few days you've been examining and analysing what, when and how you eat. Now, in your Notebook, write down the answers to these questions:

- How many eating patterns have you identified over the past week? Did you know about them already?

- Have you noticed any feelings associated with eating?

- Are there any particular times of day that trigger cravings for you?

- Are there any specific foods that trigger cravings?

- Are there certain things you do that trigger cravings?

Now do something about it

When you know what feelings make you want to eat (boredom or anxiety perhaps), you can think of other ways to make yourself feel better. If you always have a snack at four o' clock, make a point of doing something completely different at that time if you're not hungry. If it's specific foods that set you off, we'll be giving you a lot of ideas for coping with them later on, but for now, try something completely different. If there are certain activities like watching TV that make you reach for a bag of crisps, have a drink of water or take a Fat Burning Pill instead.

The Hunger Scale Danger Zone

Of course, you can't do anything about changing your eating patterns unless you're in the habit of checking the Hunger Scale. When you first start using it, the temptation is to make yourself wait until you're registering nine or ten before you eat, but that's a bad idea because you'll end up eating too quickly and that makes it hard for you to register when you're full. That's why we call nine or ten the Danger Zone and when you eat in the Danger Zone you're more likely to eat very fast and to eat fatty or sugary foods. As in real life, it's very important to proceed slowly if you're in the Danger Zone. So stick with around six or seven.

If you're still not sure exactly where you are on the scale, it may be quite a while since you really listened to your stomach.

You probably learned to over-ride the signs of hunger while you were so busy trying not to exceed your calorie allowance. As you know, Sod's Law decrees that the minute you're not allowed something you start wanting it more than anything in the universe. Especially food.

Possible signs of hunger are:

- Thinking about food when there isn't any around (especially if you can smell or taste something in particular).

- Feeling faint or headachy.

- Rumbling stomach.

- Inability to concentrate on anything but the possibility of eating.

Of course, these aren't the same for everybody and you may have your own special signals that you need to eat. It might even be a feeling you can't define. It's your job to get to know exactly what it is for you.

Challenge: The Hunger Scale Danger Zone

Continue to check, every time you eat, that you're at six or seven on the Hunger Scale.

Exercise

By now you may be getting used to the three Fat Burning Pills you're taking every day, so, if you haven't already done it, I'm going to suggest you increase your activity levels just a little bit more.

> ## Challenge: Taking a fourth Fat Burning Pill

Does that seem too much – or still too easy? If you're feeling worried about fitting it into your busy schedule, look back at the previous chapters for a few ideas you can fit around your lifestyle. Or try this:

- Set your alarm. If you have a watch or a mobile phone with an alarm function, set it to go off every two hours or so during the day.

- If it rings when you've been sitting down for a while, get up and take a Fat Burning Pill. If you've already taken four of them today, get up anyway and move around for a few minutes.

- Walk to another floor and speak to a colleague, empty the washing machine, water the plants, walk to the shops, take the dog out or whatever makes sense for you.

Remember it can mean five, ten or fifteen pennies in the Fat Jar.

> ## Challenge: First Steps Fitness
>
> Remember to keep going with these exercises – they'll make you more aware of your body, help you tone your muscles and make you feel 100% better.

DAY SIX

FIRST:

You're about to look back over your first week. Make a note in your Notebook of any loose ends – anything that hasn't quite worked for you so far and make a point today of following it through.

Today's Challenges . . .

Motivation

Giving yourself a pat on the back

Making sure you know what you want

Eating

Controlling your cutlery

Exercise

Thinking of a new Fat Burning Pill

Motivation

Challenge: Giving yourself a pat on the back
whenever you get something right

Make an effort to catch yourself doing well because that's the
best way to reinforce the good habits and weaken the negative
ones. Whenever you take a Fat Burning Pill or eat when you're
hungry and stop when you're full, give yourself a pat on the
back, literally. You can wait until nobody's looking.

Progress Check

This is the end of Week One and tomorrow you get to think
through everything you've done this week without any new
ideas to digest. You're a quarter of the way through the course
and it's time to check the Feel Good and Motivation Scales
again.

Feel Good Scale

Hopeless		Could Be Better					Very Positive		
1	2	3	4	5	6	7	8	9	10

Motivation Scale

Low									High
1	2	3	4	5	6	7	8	9	10

How are you doing?

If you didn't score as high as you'd like, what are you going
to do about it? If your Duck is still talking you down – shut it up!

(DO THIS NOW!)

Check Your Goals

Have a look at the goals for this course that you wrote down on Day One. Whether they've changed or not, write them down again.

_____

_____

_____

_____

_____

_____

Use Positive language please

Be careful what you wish for – it might come true

That's an old saying, but it comes true time and again. How often have you been close to success – in slimming or anything else – only to sabotage yourself at the last minute? We all do it, and we all agonise about it, but there's a simple explanation and an even simpler solution.

The truth is that we are comfortable with what we know. If you've been overweight for a long time, you may not like it, but you're well and truly used to it. Meena, a lady who had been doing very well on one of our courses turned up in tears on the last evening and told the group that a work colleague had asked her out for a drink.

'What's wrong with that?' we asked her.

'I'm used to my fat and jolly image,' she said. 'I didn't expect to have to re-think my lifestyle quite so quickly.'

If you're serious about changing, you'd better be sure you can cope with the consequences. The best way is to start with a reality check on the finer details of this goal of yours.

Challenge: Making sure you know what you want

If any of these questions seem irrelevant to you, or an answer doesn't immediately spring to mind, move on to the next one. Don't linger over it – the first answer is usually the truest. I've given you some ideas for the first few, but the last five questions are totally down to you. I don't want to put any ideas in your head.

? What do you want? Make it specific, 'I want to wear size 12 jeans again', or 'I want to run upstairs without getting breathless.' Make it positive as well.

_____

? When do you want it? Give yourself a time frame.

_____

? Where do you want it? Can you imagine being slimmer, fitter and healthier in your present home / job / family situation?

_____

? Who do you want it with? Do you have support from your colleagues, friends and family at the moment? Or do some of them share your problems but not your desire to change?

_____

? What would be different as a result of your achieving this goal? Could you do things you can't do now? Would it open up possibilities?

_____ ⇨

? What would achieving this do for you? How would you feel if you were slimmer, fitter and healthier?

? What would achieving this get for you? A new job? A new partner? Respect from your colleagues?

? What would achieving this give you? Only you can answer this.

? What resources do you have to accomplish this? Well, this book for a start – but what about all those qualities you noticed when you made a list of all your past achievements?

? What is it about you that will allow you to do it? What is it about you that will help you to succeed this time? Desperation – maybe! – but what about determination? Persistence? A new feeling of self-worth?

? What additional resources do you need to achieve this? Support perhaps – did you find yourself a slimming buddy? Time?

? How will you know when you've achieved it? Will it be feedback from other people? Or catching sight of yourself in the mirror and liking what you see?

? What will you be seeing, hearing, feeling, smelling, tasting? Could it be smaller clothes you're wearing? Compliments? Energy? Healthy food?

? What will you look like and sound like? We'll be helping you with this later in the book, but if you already have a clear image of that Future You it will give you a head start.

You can answer the rest of the questions without any help from me. If the answers don't immediately spring to mind, move on and answer them later.

? What will happen if you achieve this?

? What won't happen if you achieve this?

? What would you get to have or keep by *not* achieving this?

? How do you know that your goal is worth achieving?

? How will this affect your life, family, business, job, friends?

The key to success in anything, including slimming, is to be very clear about exactly what it is that you want. If you know what you want, you can practise coping with it when it happens. A lot of people who lose weight are surprised to find that life as a slim person isn't quite what they expected.

So, before we move on to Eating and Exercise, there are just a few more questions you might want to ask yourself:

- Who am I doing this for?

- What effect does my health and appearance have on other people?

- Is there anyone in my life who might be learning how to be overweight from me?

- How do my habits affect those around me?

If you come up with some useful answers, write them in your Notebook.

Eating

Challenge: Controlling your cutlery

Put down your knife and fork between bites – it will slow down your eating and give your stomach time to tell you when it's full.

Food Profile – changes over the week

It may be a bit soon, but are you noticing any changes yet in your Food Profile?

(DO THIS NOW!)

Food Check

- Do you have any persistent gaps – are there any types of food in the Foods To Focus On that you still haven't tried and don't want to?

- Do you have any persistent overloads in the Foods To Limit circle?

- Are you still eating at less than six on the Hunger Scale?

- Are you eating too quickly to register when you're full?

If your answer to any of these questions is yes, what are you going to do about it? Whether you decide to try something new, eat less of something else, or just make sure you use the Hunger Scale more regularly, make a list. You can either write your ideas down here or put them straight into your Notebook.

_____

_____

_____

Exercise

Fat Burning Pyramid

During this past week I've been asking you to build up the first two layers of your Fat Burning Pyramid. Next week I'll be introducing Feel Good Fitness, and it's very important to be starting from a solid base of frequent, brisk activity. With your First Steps exercises and four Fat Burning Pills every day, you'll be in much better shape to take on something a little more challenging.

Fat Jar Fitness

On Day Four, I asked you to think of an everyday task that could also be a Fat Burning Pill. I don't know if you came up with something and tried it out – from my experience most people settle for one kind of Fat Jar activity and stick with it – but I don't want you to settle down too soon – Lighten Up is about getting out of your box and stretching your comfort zone.

Challenge: Thinking of a new Fat Burning Pill

Think of a new Fat Burning Pill (up to fifteen minutes of brisk exercise), but make it something you haven't done before and do it today, as part of your Fat Jar Fitness. If you normally have a short walk, then this time climb some stairs or dance to your favourite song.

DAY SEVEN

There are no new exercises, challenges or targets for Day Seven. You've had a lot of new ideas to take in this week, and so today is all about giving yourself a chance to reflect on what you've been learning.

Take it easy, congratulate yourself on how well you've been doing, and have a great day!

Week Two

WEEK TWO STARTER

FIRST: _____

Review your first six days of Lighten Up by reading quickly through your Notebook, day by day. It's important to do this before you answer the next list of questions.

(DO THIS NOW!)

Of the techniques I learned, what do I *want* to keep doing, do more of or do better?

	Keep doing	Do more of	Try again
Motivation			
Dealing with my inner critic (or Duck) and talking to myself positively every day			
Giving myself credit when I get something right			⇨

	Keep doing	Do more of	Try again
Using my Notebook to keep track of my progress			
Eating			
Filling in the Food Profile			
Eating types of food I've never eaten before			
Eating more fruit and vegetables			
Drinking plenty of water every day			
Identifying and getting rid of poor eating habits			
Eating by the Hunger Scale			
Slowing down my eating			
Exercise			
Using the Exercise Wheel to see how active I am			
Incorporating Fat Jar Fitness sessions into my daily life			
Fitting in First Steps exercises			

Most slimming programmes work against all your natural instincts and inclinations. Lighten Up, on the other hand, works *with* you – but it won't work *for* you. It's *your* input and commitment that will make the difference.

Eating

Remember to keep filling in the Food Profiles this week.

Exercise

You've already started to build the foundations of your Fat Burning Pyramid, and this week it's time to move up to the next level – Feel Good Fitness. I'll go into more detail on Day One, but all you need to know for now is that you should aim to do three Feel Good Fitness sessions this week. So decide right now on which days you're going to fit them in, and write them in both your Notebook *and* your diary as you would any other important appointment – that way you're more likely to stick to them.

Feel Good Fitness is the top layer of your Fat Burning Pyramid, and it's different because:

- The sessions are longer.

- You'll need to wear appropriate and comfortable (but not necessarily expensive) clothes, which allow free movement – trainers optional.

- It's more strenuous, so you'll be hot and sweaty and probably need to shower.

A lot of the most obvious kinds of Feel Good Fitness – such as using a step machine or resistance training with weights – involve things like joining a gym or at least finding a sports centre, but that really doesn't have to be the case. There's lots of Feel Good Fitness you can do from home, without making any major financial commitment or outlay, so don't panic!

In Chapter 6 you'll find a great basic fitness programme you can do at home, and we've also included some suggestions for fitness videos and inexpensive fitness equipment, so have a look there if you need inspiration.

If you're just getting started on an exercise programme, it's always a good idea to go for something you think will be fun. If there's anything you've enjoyed doing in the past, that's a good place to start.

If you've never had one single good exercise experience in the past, make a fresh start. Pick something you've always fancied and give it a go.

Remember, whatever you chose, to include time for warming up and cooling down. The stretches in Chapter 6 can be used for this. And see the note about warming up and cooling down on page 252 of Chapter 5.

DO THIS NOW!

- What are your current activity levels – including both Fat Jar Fitness and Feel Good Fitness?

- What's your previous experience of exercising been like (assuming you have some)?

- What are your likes and dislikes – is there anything you've tried before and hated? Or loved? Do you like team sports? Solitary walks? Swimming? Tennis? Jogging? Cycling? Rowing? Trampolining? Aerobics? Dancing?

- How successful have you been with exercise routines in the past?

- What's your basic attitude towards exercise? Do you think it's necessary? Or fun? Or unnecessary? (Some people think diet alone can do it.)

- What are the common factors in the activities you've enjoyed before?

  o Being alone?

  o Competing with other people?

  o Sharing activities – exercise with a social side?

  o Having an audience?

- ○ Being outdoors or indoors?

- ○ Exercising in the morning or evening?

- ○ Music? Style? Setting?

- ○ _____ ?

- ○ _____ ?

- What are the common factors, if any, in the activities you haven't enjoyed – the ones you gave up on?

  - ○ _____ ?

  - ○ _____ ?

Use this to help you choose the Feel Good Fitness activities that will work for you.

Bearing in mind the list of criteria you've just drawn up, consider the (almost limitless) possibilities for Feel Good Fitness exercise, but be practical – the best kind of exercise for you may well be whatever you would find it easiest to do on a regular basis. There are plenty of different activities to choose from – and the great thing is that most of them actively encourage beginners to sign up. Here are a few ideas:

Abseiling	Hockey	Sprinting
Aerobics	Hurdling	Step classes
Badminton	Jogging	Swimming
Ballet	Karate	Tai Chi
Belly dancing	Kick boxing	Tango dancing
Canoeing	Netball	Tennis
Climbing	Orienteering	Triathlon
Cycling	Potholing	Weightlifting
Football	Rowing	Windsurfing
Hash running	Rugby	
Hiking	Salsa dancing	

And don't worry, you can do lots of these (for instance, aerobics, kick boxing, salsa, step) from home if you get a fitness video and clear a bit of space in front of the TV.

A reminder about Fat Jar Fitness

Remember that incorporating Feel Good Fitness into your life doesn't mean giving up on Fat Jar Fitness. In fact, you should be trying to work in four or five Fat Jar breaks a day this week.

Checklist

1. Set up your Notebook for the next six days so that each day is ready for you. Get your Food Profile copied or drawn in, and the Exercise Wheel as well if you plan to continue using it.

2. Make sure you have:

   - Trainers – you're going to move up to the Feel Good Fitness level of your Fat Burning Pyramid so you'll need a good pair. They're also useful for Fat Jar Fitness.

   - Healthy food to eat at home and carry with you when you go out.

   - Your bottle of water.

DAY ONE

FIRST:

Put yourself in a positive frame of mind by doing a First Steps session before you read any further. You can count it as one of your First Steps sessions for today.

Today's challenges . . .

Motivation

Polishing up your self-image

Eating

Eating without distractions

Exercise

Raising your exercise level

Motivation

Slimming From The Head Down

If you want to change your body, the best place to start is in your mind. If you treat your body like a machine and try to get results with the 'calories in must be less than calories out' approach, it won't work. Your mind will sabotage your body every time unless you engage your brain right at the start of your slimming programme.

A well-known glossy woman's magazine ran an interesting experiment with a group of women who were all asked to draw their outline on a piece of paper. One woman's outline had enormous thighs, several of them looked like Teletubbies and all of the sketches were plump to say the least. Yet these were all normal, well-proportioned women with dress sizes between ten and fourteen.

Most women, and an increasing number of men, see themselves as larger than they really are. If I were to ask you to draw your own outline and show it to a friend, would they know it was you?

(DO THIS NOW!)

Slimming Scale

Quickly scan through this list and tick all the words that apply to you.

Achiever	Bingeing	Comfortable
Anti-Social	Bonny	Confident
Anxious	Bony	Controlled
Ashamed	Boring	Controlling
Athletic	Boyish	Couch Potato
Attractive	Bulging	Cuddly
Beautiful	Cheating	Curvy

Datable	Funny	Self-esteem high
Depressing	Girly	Self-esteem low
Deprived	Gross	Sensual
Deserving	Handsome	Sexy
Determined	Happy	Shapely
Dieter	Hopeless	Skinny
Difficult	Huggable	Slim
Disciplined	Hunky	Slow
Dynamic	Image-conscious	Sluggish
Elegant	Interesting	Stable
Embarrassed	Jolly	Starving
Empty	Lonely	Strong
Energetic	Lovely	Strong-willed
Excessive	Magnetic	Successful
Excitable	Manly	Suffering
Exhausted	Masculine	Thin
Failure	Monstrous	Tired
Fascinating	Motherly	Trendy
Fashionable	Motivated	Ugly
Fat	Muscular	Unattractive
Fatherly	Obsessive	Uncontrolled
Feminine	Old	Unfit
Firm	Party animal	Voluptuous
Fit	Pleasure seeker	Weighty
Fit In	Plump	Wimp
Flirty	Popular	Womanly
Floppy	Powerful	Worried
Frumpy	Round	
Friendly	Self Deluding	

This checklist will give you a pretty good indication of how much confidence you have in your ability to be a slim person.

Write down the words you've ticked into lists of positive words and negative words. Take a look at the negative list. If you continue to live with those feelings about yourself they will slow down your slimming programme. Just for now, leave them on the page and remind yourself they are just words. We'll show you how to deal with them later.

Next look at the positive list and copy that into your Notebook. How do those words make you feel? If you didn't tick *any* positive words, look through the list again and pick three *that you would like to believe*. It doesn't matter if you really do believe them or not, we'll work on that later.

Challenge: Polishing up your self-image

- Write two or three of the positive words from the list above (the ones you believe or the ones you'd like to believe) on a Post-It note (a large one!). Stick it on your bathroom mirror or somewhere you'll see it every day.

- In your Notebook, write a description of the way you think you look right now. Just a paragraph will do. Describe your clothes, your posture, your expression, your hair, your weight and shape. Now write another description of you, but imagine you are writing it exactly a year from now, picturing the way you'll be looking then. What do you see? I hope the second description will be a much more positive one. If it's not, tear it up, or cross it out, and start again.

Eating

Food Rules

Why am I not telling you exactly what to eat? Because I don't know you well enough to do that. What Lighten Up does do is provide the three tools you need to make the right choices for you:

- The Hunger Scale helps tell you when to eat.

- The Foods To Focus On circle suggests what types of food to eat

- Eating slowly and paying attention to how you feel will help you decide *how much* to eat.

Lighten Up isn't about restricting what you eat. It's about eating what you need and getting as much pleasure as possible out of it. That means eating *slowly* – always taking care to put really good food into your body. When you start to think what your body needs and what will feel good inside you, it will be easier to eat well.

So, next time you eat, ask yourself these questions:

- Can I taste the different ingredients – what is the strongest flavour?
- What do I like about the texture of this food?
- Does it smell as good as, or better than, it tastes?
- How does it make me feel while I'm eating it?
- At what point do I stop feeling hungry?
- How does it feel to leave food on the plate?
- Do I feel as good after I've eaten as I did before – or better?
- Is there a point during the meal when I start to feel as though I can't be bothered to finish?
- While I'm eating this meal, am I thinking about what I'm going to eat later in the day, or even tomorrow morning?

Food Profile Reminder

Fill in your Food Profile for another week. It will really help you to get a better feel for:

● What you need to eat.

● What you're actually eating.

● How much progress you're making.

Challenge: Eating without distractions

Eat one meal today without doing anything else at the same time. When you eat that meal, you'll have plenty of time to focus on the food you're eating and what it's doing for you, and you'll be much more likely to stop when you're full.

Exercise

Back in the Week Two Starter you chose the three days this week when you're going to start incorporating some Feel Good Fitness. Now's the time to get going and it's important to know whether you're exercising at the right level when you're doing Fat Jar Fitness or Feel Good Fitness.

You can use a heart rate monitor of course, but the easiest way to hit the right level is to get to know yourself better and start becoming more aware of your breathing. You can do that using the Borg Scale:

The Borg Scale									
	First Steps Fitness		**Fat Jar Fitness**			**Feel Good Fitness**			
1	2	3	4	5	6	7	8	9	10
			Gentle to brisk exercise. Breathing faster than normal.			Comfortable exercise. **Deep, fast breathing**. Really feel your body working, burning *fat*. Can talk (carry on a conversation) whilst exercising.		Out of breath. Really hard work. Not enjoying it. Burning sugar.	

Feel Good Fitness is quite easy to define – between six and eight is about right and you'll know when you hit nine or ten because at that level you *won't* be feeling good (unless you're already pretty fit and are training in a very specific way).

There's more of an overlap between First Steps Fitness and Fat Jar Fitness however – it's not a clear division between levels three and four as it appears on the scale. A lot depends on you and your current level of personal fitness. As you get used to being more active, you will find you can do things like walking up a flight of stairs without any breathlessness at all – something you may not have thought possible before.

Challenge: Raising your exercise levels

- Is today one of your Feel Good Fitness days? If so, make sure you make time for it, and make sure you've chosen something you'll enjoy.

- If today isn't one of your Feel Good Fitness days, fit in an extra Fat Jar Fitness session instead.

DAY TWO

FIRST:

Make a list in your Notebook of the positive changes you've made so far. It doesn't matter if they are tiny, or if there are only one or two. Write them down and congratulate yourself.

Today's challenges . . .

Motivation

Recognising hunger

Eating

Eating fruit you've never tried before

Keeping up the Food Profiles

Exercise

Raising your exercise levels

Motivation

Awareness, awareness, awareness

If you want to succeed and achieve your Lighten Up goals, you need to:

- Notice what *doesn't* work so you can substitute something that does. If eating quickly, for example, is making it hard to stop when you're full, then eat slowly.

- Notice what *does* work so that you can do even more of it. If doing some First Steps exercises takes your mind off the biscuits, then use your First Steps programme to distract you from sweet snacks when you aren't hungry.

You have probably spent enough time in the past judging yourself and blaming yourself when things go wrong. You'll get better results if you simply notice what's happening, what makes you eat, what makes you avoid exercise and what your inner critic or Duck is telling you about failure.

You can use your Notebook to help you with this personal detective work. You will get better information about yourself from the things you write in your Notebook than you would get from anyone else because you are free to tell it to yourself like it really is. If you're honest enough to do that, you'll soon be able to draw your own conclusions about what you can change. Remember: *it works much better if you write it down*!

Challenge: Recognising hunger

Write this list of basic questions in your notebook:

- Am I genuinely hungry?

- Why am I eating if I'm not hungry?

- How do I feel *before* I eat when I'm not hungry?

- How do I feel *after* I eat when I'm not hungry?

- What sort of food do I eat when I'm not hungry?

Ask yourself these questions every time you eat – or want to eat – today. Jot down the answers. You'll start to see some patterns emerging (and of course if you find you're genuinely not hungry, then think twice before putting food in your mouth).

If you ask yourself the same questions every day this week, you'll learn a lot about your eating patterns – and getting to know your own eating patterns makes it so much easier to interrupt and change them. When you know your weak points, you can decide where and how to intervene and do things differently.

Eating

Food for life

The idea that fruit and vegetables are good for us is probably less controversial than any other piece of nutritional information. In spite of that, most people in the UK don't even get close to their Five a Day target. Unless you count chips of course.

Fruit and vegetables are so nutritious that eating enough of them should make it unnecessary to take supplements. The fresher they are, the more of their goodness (and flavour) they retain.

Challenge: Eating fruit you've never tried before

Try some fresh fruit you don't normally eat, for example:

Gooseberries	Kiwi fruit	Figs
Loganberries	Lychees	Apricots
Blueberries	Mangoes	Cherries
Grapefruit	Passion-fruit	Plums
Pineapple	Pomegranates	Melon

They don't have to be expensive, and there's now a huge range available all year round.

Challenge: Keeping up the Food Profile

Remember to fill out your Food Profile today.

Exercise

Feel Good Fitness can be either aerobic exercise (cardiovascular fitness – which can be measured on the Borg Scale) or resistance training (flexing your muscles against some resistance).

What will Feel Good Fitness do for me?

- Aerobic/cardiovascular exercise raises your pulse and breathing rate and increases the efficiency of your heart and lungs so that blood and oxygen is supplied more efficiently.

- Resistance work will strengthen your muscles and trained muscles burn fat even when you aren't using them. (Note, your First Steps count as resistance work so you've actually already started.)

- Exercise helps you regulate your appetite.*

- It makes you feel good.

Remember, it's important to find a Feel Good Fitness activity you enjoy. To get the most benefit, combine some cardiovascular work and some resistance work (see Chapter 6 for the Lighten Up Home Exercise Programme).

Challenge: Raising your exercise levels

- Is today one of your Feel Good Fitness days? If so, make sure you make time for it, and make sure you've chosen something you'll enjoy.

- If today isn't one of your Feel Good Fitness days, try to fit in an extra Fat Jar Fitness session instead.

---

*Brookhaven National Laboratory, New York 2001.

DAY THREE

FIRST: _____

Where are you on the Motivation and Feel Good scales at the moment? By Week Two most people are a little higher up the scale than where they started. If you're stuck, do something about it before you move on. Remember what went well for you yesterday. Even if you snacked a lot and missed some of your Fat Burning Pills and First Steps sessions, give yourself credit for things you did do. That extra piece of fruit perhaps, taking a walk, using the Hunger Scale or eating more slowly.

And you could look back in your Notebook at that description you wrote of yourself, a year into the future and see how much better and how much more confident that makes you feel as well.

Today's challenges . . .

Motivation

Think Before You Eat

Eating

The Rainbow Theory

Exercise

Blending your First Steps Fitness and Fat Jar Fitness into your daily routine

Motivation

Today we're going to start with one of the most important Lighten Up techniques – Think Before You Eat. It's incredibly easy – in fact, for slim people it's instinctive – and it can be second nature for you too, if you take a little time to practise.

Think Before You Eat

Next time you're in the mood for eating, check the Hunger Scale. If you're registering at least six or seven, find a quiet place where you can relax, undisturbed, to decide what you really want to eat.

When you're ready, sit down with your eyes closed and do the following:

(DO THIS NOW!)

Think Before You Eat

- Now that you've decided you're ready to eat, what do you fancy? A double hamburger with melted cheese and bacon? A banana and peanut butter sandwich? A slice of chocolate cake? A tuna salad? Some foods are easy to imagine (think of biting into a lemon), but if whatever you're thinking of doesn't tickle your tastebuds you're either not really hungry after all or you don't really want that particular food.

- When you've made your choice, imagine eating it. Taste it, smell it, feel it in your mouth and swallow it. How will you feel half an hour, and then an hour afterwards? Will it make you feel bloated? Will it give you energy? Or are you more likely to need a nap? Will it be used up in your body or will it be stored somewhere?

- If you still feel like eating it, make it the first item on your mental list. If not, forget it.

- Now think of something else you might want to eat and run through the same process, smelling, tasting and thinking how you'll feel afterwards.

- Carry on picking items from your imaginary menu and checking them out in your imagination.

- When you have two or three possible choices on your mental list, make your final selection. Which one would you actually choose?

Think Before You Eat becomes automatic quite quickly and you'll soon be running through it in seconds. If you take time to listen to your body by running this process, you'll be surprised at the healthy messages you start to get.

There are two questions which often arise:

Q: If my body knows I need Food To Focus On, why do I usually end up eating Food To Limit?

A: Your body will tell you what you need, but your brain will tell you what you want. Mostly we listen to our brains instead of our bodies.

Q: Why can't my brain and body agree on this?

A: As you grew up, you taught your brain to over-ride your body's demands – and there are a lot of social situations where this arrangement works well. However, when it comes to eating and exercising, you want to get your body and brain working together as a team again. It's just a matter of practice.

Challenge: Think Before You Eat

Do this every time you have a meal today.

Eating

The Food Profile diagram you have been using was designed to give you information at a glance and your eating challenge today is a visual one too.

The Rainbow Theory

You know that the freshest possible fruit and vegetables are your best basic eating essentials, and if you're not sure which ones to go for, the Rainbow Theory is a good approximate guide to getting the right balance.

Fruit and vegetable colours are an indication of the nutrients they contain and the most highly coloured foods are sometimes the most nutritious. For instance:

Red	Orange	Yellow	Green/Blue	Brown	White
Tomatoes	Carrots	Corn	Spinach	Grains	Calcium rich
Beetroot	Pumpkin	Lemons	Broccoli		foods like:
Raspberries	Apricots	Bananas	Blueberries		milk,
Strawberries	Oranges	Peaches	Cucumber		yoghurt, fish

This isn't meant to be precise, but a good rule of thumb is that if you go for a good mix of colours in your food, you've got a good chance of getting the variety you need.

Challenge: The Rainbow Theory

Incorporate a new vegetable into your diet – but make it a different colour from the ones you'd normally choose.

Exercise

Two First Steps sessions and three Fat Burning Pills in the Fat Jar sounds like a lot, but these activities are designed to be woven into your life – you shouldn't have to take significant time out for them. Most of us have moments during the day when we're waiting for the kettle to boil, or the children to get ready for school, or the computer to log on to the internet – perfect times for a First Steps session. And the Fat Burning Pills are designed either to get you somewhere or to get something done.

Challenge: Blending First Steps and Fat Jar Fitness into your daily routine

As well as your Feel Good Fitness, see how many of your First Steps sessions and Fat Jar breaks you can fit into other daily activities.

DAY FOUR

FIRST:

Before you start reading today, think about your next Feel Good Fitness session. Do you know when it will be and what you'll be doing? Have you remembered to write it in your Notebook and appointments diary?

Today's challenges . . .

Motivation

Daydreaming yourself thin

Think Before You Eat

Eating

Drinking enough water

Eliminating two poor habits

Exercise

Developing a more active lifestyle

Motivation

Are you ready for your new role?

Remember the Oscar you accepted back on Day Three of Week One for that overweight role you've played so brilliantly for so long? Well, you're getting ready now for your new role as a slim person.

Can you really use your mind to change your shape? Of course you can. There's a drama school in Hollywood which helps actors fit their roles by changing their body shape. They use the kind of visualisation you're about do next and it works like this: if you constantly picture yourself as a slim person, you are much more likely to make the eating and exercise choices a slim person would make.

(DO THIS NOW!)

The Future You
(with thanks to Paul McKenna)

You might like to record this visualisation so that you can listen to yourself talking you through it. Also, there are versions of it on the Lighten Up tape. This is a good one to do with your Slimming Buddy if you have one. Having someone to talk you through it can help a lot.

- Choose a time and place when you aren't going to be interrupted. Stand up, close your eyes and take a couple of deep breaths. Check that you are relaxed from your shoulders right down to your toes.

- Think about your front door. Have you got a clear picture of it? Or do you just have a feeling that it's there? Maybe you can hear the key as you put it in the lock, or the sounds of the street. Imagine you're standing right in front of it, about to put your key in the lock and step inside.   ⇨

- As the door opens, you can see an image of yourself at some time in the future, standing there in the hallway.

- The Future You is slimmer, fitter and healthier. You are just the way you want to be, at your ideal size, glowing with health and feeling confident and happy.

- See how much detail you notice: your clothes, your hair, your skin, the way you are standing and the expression on your face.

- The Future You is close enough to touch and the image is strong and vivid. If it's not as clear as you'd like at first, you'll find that practice will make perfect.

- For now, just see as much as you can and picture your Future You turning around so you can see yourself from every angle.

- When the Future You has gone full circle and is facing away from you again, step forward into yourself. Walk right into your new, slim, fit and healthy body, as if you're putting on a new skin.

- Notice how you feel when you're doing this. Light-hearted and light-headed perhaps? Graceful and free? Or just comfortable in yourself?

- When you get that good feeling, remember it. Then run through the Future You visualisation again. Make it stronger this time and see how much better you can look as your confidence increases.

Of course, it doesn't have to be your front door that you're walking through – we chose it because it's easy to imagine for most people. You might prefer your garden gate, a cricket pitch, the finishing line at the marathon, a catwalk at a fashion show, a stage at Glastonbury, or walking down the aisle – it's up to you.

If you don't get much time to yourself, you can still check out the Future You, even if you are sitting on the train, for example, or waiting in a queue. But it's best to start by creating some personal space until you really get the hang of it.

Challenge: Daydreaming yourself thin

Start daydreaming several times a day about what you'll look like when you're slim.

Challenge: Think Before You Eat

Make sure you're continuing to use Think Before You Eat.

Eating

I'm starting the Eating part of today's programme by focusing on what you drink rather than what you eat. From looking at the Food Profile you can see that we've put water in a category by itself, not because it's a food group – most food has water in it – but because it's so important.

Water

In spite of the publicity for drinking plenty of water, and even in spite of the fact that a bottle of water appears to be a fashion accessory, most of us don't drink enough. The British Nutrition Foundation recommends more than two litres a day of *fluid* although of course this doesn't take into account body size, temperature and activity levels. I suggest you go for around two litres a day of *water*, not counting any other drinks you may have (some of which, especially coffee, tea and alcohol, will have a diuretic effect anyway).

Remember:

- Drinking plenty of water helps your digestive system, liver and kidneys, to work efficiently.

- You can check for dehydration by checking the colour of your urine – it should be pale straw coloured, not dark yellow.

- Drinking plenty of water means you're less likely to confuse hunger and thirst, so you won't end up eating when you really need to drink. In fact, having a glass of water may be a good substitute for eating if you're trying to break a particular pattern, like snacking to stay awake while you work. You could sip water instead.

Challenge: Drinking enough water

If you aren't already drinking plenty of water, fill up a glass or a bottle and start now, and make sure you drink two litres today. It might sound a lot, but it's only four small-size bottles of water over the whole day.

Now we'll move on to eating patterns. How many of your overeating habits have you nailed down and eliminated? When are you going to tackle the rest? And what are you going to do instead?

DO THIS NOW!

Common Eating Patterns

I'm sure you can add some of your own!

- Eating something sweet mid-morning because you missed breakfast.

- Snacking to stay awake at your desk.

- Going for a chocolate bar to keep you going through the afternoon energy dip.

- Heading straight for the fridge when you get in from work.

- Nibbling popcorn or crisps while you watch TV.

- Getting late night kebabs and curries after you've been for a drink.

- Having a biscuit or two with a cup of tea.

- _____

- _____

- _____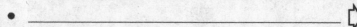

In your Notebook, list the negative eating habits you still want to get rid of and what you plan to do about them.

Then list your good eating habits and how you can build on them.

Challenge: Eliminating two poor habits

Choose two patterns from your list, and make a promise to yourself not to indulge either of them today . Remember to write them down in your Notebook.

Exercise

(DO THIS NOW!)

Pick Your Problem

Here are some of the problems people mention when I ask them
why they don't keep going with their Feel Good Fitness
programme. Do any of them apply to you?

- I keep getting injured.

- I keep getting ill.

- I never quite reach the standard I want.

- I'm not winning often enough to stay motivated.

- I don't have enough time.

- I don't have the money.

- The family gets in the way.

- Work gets in the way.

- I don't have the facilities.

- I don't have the support.

- I'm getting too old.

- I keep getting side-tracked.

- _____

- _____

- _____

If you ticked any of those or came up with some of your own, I
have another question for you. What are you going to do about
it?

Feel Good Fitness

Be realistic. What are you willing to give up in order to get some Feel Good Fitness into your life? Figure out where you have some leeway and where you don't. If your life revolves around work, or children (or both), you may have to be creative about when, where and how you fit in your exercise sessions. It's definitely getting easier though. Health and fitness clubs are open early and late and there are more of them around, so before or after work sessions are possible options – as are lunchbreak workouts. And lots of places have crèches and children's activities where ten years ago there were none.

So, ask yourself: what am I prepared to give up in order to exercise?

- Watching television?   • _____
- Lying in bed?   • _____
- Going to the pub?   • _____
- Shopping?   • _____
- Staying late at work?   • _____

When you've decided how much time you can free up for exercise, you're ready to make a start. Remember to plan in your warm-up and cool-down time as well as your showering, travelling and changing time. This is why, if time is short, it's a good idea to do something that is close at hand and doesn't involve elaborate arrangements. If you're particularly busy this week, look at Chapter 6 for some ideas of exercise programmes you can do at home.

Challenge: Developing a more active lifestyle

Look at your Exercise Wheel and ask yourself: How am I going to fit a more active lifestyle into the same twenty-four hours?

DAY FIVE

FIRST: _____

Check where you are on the Motivation and Feel Good Scales and write it down in your Notebook before you start reading about today. Quantifying how you feel is a very useful habit to get into because it stops you turning into a boiled frog.*

Today's challenges . . .

Motivation

Making up an inspiring Affirmation

Reviewing your goal

Eating

Controlling your cravings

Experimenting with some new recipes

Exercise

Checking your Borg Scale level

---

* Apparently if you try and put a frog in hot water it will jump out, but if you put it into cold water and gradually bring it to the boil it ends up as a Eurosnack. Demotivation, especially in the middle of a slimming programme, can creep up on you. If you don't notice how far you've slipped back until halfway through the fridge contents, it may be too late.

Motivation

Three steps to success

Put these ideas together, take them a little bit further and you'll have a series of stepping-stones that will take you nearer your goal.

1. Thinking positive

Yes, we've already talked about using positive language when you talk to yourself. This is just a reminder. Saying 'I'm getting slimmer,' instead of 'I must lose weight', makes you feel better, and the better you feel the more likely you are to take positive action. Apart from a quick jump-start session with the Scrooge exercise, you're more likely to upgrade your eating and exercise habits if you're feeling good. Feeling depressed about your weight creates inertia not energy. It's energy you need because energy burns calories and builds muscle (which in turn burns even more calories).

2. Using Affirmations

Remember the two lists of positive and negative words you chose on Day One of this week (page 100) to describe yourself in the Slimming Scale? I suggested you post up three positive ones in a place where you could look at them regularly, such as on the bathroom mirror.

If you now put these words into a sentence (with a positive spin to it of course) you get an Affirmation. Will Affirmations make you lose weight? Well, no, they won't, not by themselves. But this is about re-writing and if necessary re-wiring your entire inner dialogue (the way you talk to yourself). It's the first step to building your new belief that you can be slim.

3. Asking good questions

If you ask yourself critical questions: 'Why do I always eat too much? . . . Why do I keep putting on weight?' you will get negative answers: 'Because you're greedy . . . because you're lazy . . . because you haven't got any will power . . . because you've got a slow metabolism.' In fact, when you're talking to yourself, you'll find that, in general, questions starting with 'why' are not very helpful.

On the other hand, if you ask yourself constructive questions like 'What kind of Feel Good Fitness might I enjoy?' or 'Where can I fit in another First Steps session?', your brain will look for constructive, practical answers.

Challenge: Making up an inspiring Affirmation

Make up an inspiring Affirmation and put it somewhere you can see it.

If you can't think of anything right now, how about:

- 'I'm getting slimmer, fitter and healthier'
- 'I'm looking and feeling slimmer, sexier and stronger'
- 'I'm feeling confident about myself'

Challenge: Reviewing Your Goals

Now it's time to revisit your goals. Have they changed since Week One on page 42? Write them down in your Notebook again – sometimes just writing them down can make a difference.

- Do you expect to achieve them? On a Confidence Scale of one to ten how likely is it that you'll achieve your goals?

- Can you see yourself looking like and feeling like the person you want to be?

If you sometimes read your goal statement and feel sceptical, practise your visualisation and your affirmations separately until each goal starts to feel more realistic. Be patient and persistent, Or accept yourself the way you are.

The choice is yours

Eating

Before you read this section, flip back and have a quick look at the Food Profile diagram on page 22 – in particular the sections marked 'Complex Carbohydrates' and 'Simple Carbohydrates'. It is important to know the difference.

Simple Carbohydrates

Carbohydrates can be simple or complex and both provide us with energy. Simple carbohydrates – or sugar – are released very quickly into the bloodstream and if the body can't use them immediately they eventually end up stored as fat.

Complex Carbohydrates

Complex Carbohydrates such as wholemeal bread, pasta, brown rice and potatoes are absorbed more slowly because they take a little longer to digest. That gives the body more time to turn them gradually into energy.

Knowing the difference

It's sometimes hard to tell the difference between simple and complex carbohydrates. The simplest method is probably to use the 'No Label' shopping rule I mentioned before because:

- There's generally less sugar in natural foods and although some fruit and vegetables are high in simple carbohydrates, they're still a better choice than sweets because of their high vitamin, mineral and fibre content.

- Much of our food is processed and refined and contains 'hidden' sugar which is added to make it taste better. 'Low fat' labelled slimming foods often contain sugar for just this reason.

Challenge: Controlling your cravings

Next time you feel your energy dip and want to reach for a chocolate bar (this happens to a lot of us mid-afternoon) pause for a moment. Ask yourself if something from Foods To Focus On might keep you going for longer. Think before you eat to get an idea of what your body really needs.

Challenge: Experimenting with some new recipes

Try something new from the recipes in Chapter 8.

Exercise

You should by now be incorporating exercise from all three levels of the Fat Burning Pyramid into your week.

Challenge: Checking your Borg Scale level

Check where you are on the Borg Scale (page 105) when you are exercising at any level on the Fat Burning Pyramid.

DAY SIX

FIRST: _____

Very often, at the beginning of the day, I ask you to check where you are on one of the many Lighten Up scales. That's because it's a good idea to know where you are before you start.

Today I want you to think about where you would be right now on a Self-Esteem scale (one is low and ten is high, as usual).

Today's challenges . . .

Motivation

Raising your self-esteem

Asking yourself helpful questions

Eating

Cutting out all confectionery for a day

The Food Profile

Exercise

Varying your First Steps sessions

Increasing your Fat Jar Fitness

Checking your Feel Good Fitness levels

Motivation

You'll have noticed that for the past two weeks I've been giving you more questions than answers.

The reason is simple: Lighten Up is about getting to know yourself better. Unless you know why you have a problem with your body, you won't be able to solve that problem in the long term. Once you know *why* you aren't eating and exercising well enough to keep you slim, you can do something about it. Then there'll be nothing to stop you making healthy eating and exercise part of your life. Healthy eating and exercise won't be something you have to do – they will be part of who you are.

So keep asking questions. For example:

- Do you find that most days you have emotions you don't like?

- What are they?

- Do they often stem from the questions you ask yourself?

- Can you think what sort of questions they might be? (Here's a clue – they often start with 'Why'.)

If you can substitute positive questions for those negative ones, you'll start to get results. For instance:

- 'What's great about what I am doing?'

- 'How can I become slimmer right now?'

- 'What can I do that will start me on the road to becoming slimmer?'

- 'What do I need to do to make sure that I have a great day?'

I don't know what your own personal unwanted emotions might be, but I can tell you about the one that seems to be most often linked with weight problems. You can probably guess what it is because I've hinted at it already – it's low self-esteem.

If you have some of that, I'm going to help you get rid of it. It's not helpful, it's not realistic and it's not going to help you lose weight. If you sometimes feel bad about yourself, you may find you're tempted to over-eat, under-exercise and generally neglect yourself. I know you'd like to lose these feelings, so here's the plan:

DO THIS NOW!

Self-Esteem Step One – De-bug your system

If you work on a computer, you probably save your valuable, creative files, delete all the rubbish and check for bugs. Our brains are the most sophisticated computers we'll ever own, but we don't look after them as well as we look after our PCs. However, did you know you can programme your brain to boost your self-esteem?

- Use the right programming language and be positive when you talk to yourself. Instead of saying 'I shouldn't eat so much', 'I mustn't be so lazy', 'I can't cope under pressure', use phrases such as 'I can eat healthy food', 'I will take regular exercise', 'I am getting more confident'.

- Congratulate yourself when things go right – even little things like fitting your First Steps exercises into a busy day or making time for a healthy lunch.

- If something is bothering you, whether it's a person, an incident, or something you did or didn't do, acknowledge it, learn from it and then delete it. It's taking up valuable mind space and undermining your self-esteem.

- Before you go to sleep, think of six things that made you feel good during the day – particularly the things you did to nourish and strengthen yourself. It could be a walk you took, a meal that energised you instead of making you feel sluggish and overfull, or a body cue you took notice of (you needed to move, or rest or drink some water perhaps).

- If something's bothering you, ask yourself some questions about it. Make sure you phrase those questions positively – don't ask yourself 'Why am I such a failure?' just before you close your eyes. Instead ask 'How can I be fitter, healthier, happier?'

Step One is about having a positive attitude to yourself all the time. Step Two in the Self-Esteem programme is about giving yourself the best possible start on a daily basis.

DO THIS NOW!

Self-Esteem Step Two – Start the day right

I assume you're reading this in the morning and mornings often seem to be a bad time for a lot of people. But if you start off sluggishly, the negative mood can slow you down. It can drive you to doughnuts instead of a healthy breakfast, or send you to the pub at lunchtime when you meant to go for a swim.

Put yourself in a positive frame of mind first thing by asking yourself these questions:

- If I went to sleep last night with a question in mind, am I any closer to an answer now? (If you don't have that answer yet, don't chase it. Wait until it comes.)

- What am I happy about in my life? (These don't have to be major public triumphs; small happinesses count.)

- What am I excited about?

- What am I proud of?

- What am I grateful for?
- What am I committed to?

You could even add these questions to the collection of inspirational notes on your dressing table – or put them by your bed and read them through before you get out of bed tomorrow.

Challenge: Raising your Self-Esteem

Before you go any further, read through the Self-Esteem exercises again.

Challenge: Asking yourself helpful questions

Every time your inner critic or Duck asks you a question today ('Why am I so useless', for example), stop and turn it into a positive one – e.g. 'How can I take my next Fat Burning Pill?'

Eating

Sugar

There's a book called *Pure white and deadly** and no, it's not about cocaine. It's about sugar – or simple carbohydrates.

Sugar triggers a release of chemicals in the brain that make you feel good. Because it's absorbed so quickly into the bloodstream you'll feel that hit very soon after you've eaten your chocolate or drunk your cola.

No wonder then that so many of us crave sweet things. But if you want to lose weight, cutting down on your intake of sugary sweets and chocolate is a great way to do it – and you don't need sweets and chocolates for a healthy diet anyway.

Challenge: Cutting out all confectionery for a day

Try cutting out all confectionery – just for today. It's not permanent –as we've said before, Lighten Up is about making choices not eliminating them - but it's a useful experiment. I want you to notice how you feel without it, and to remember that you have a choice about whether you eat it or not. If you manage OK without sweets and chocolate today, do you have to go back to eating them tomorrow? It's up to you. And how about cutting out all sweet things for a day, including sugar in tea and coffee?

Challenge: The Food Profile

Make sure you fill out the Food Profile.

**Pure, white and deadly: the problem of sugar* by John Yudkin, Davis-Poynter Ltd.

Exercise

The Fat Burning Pyramid

The basic structure of your Fat Burning Pyramid should be pretty much in place by now – you're just fine tuning it.

First Steps

This is the point in the programme where you may be feeling that, yes, the First Steps sessions are easy – you know them so well that you can do them almost without thinking, while you're making a cup of tea, or deciding what to wear, or even while you're chatting to somebody in the kitchen. After all, your family and friends are probably getting used to this by now. Maybe they're even joining in!

Challenge: Varying your First Steps sessions

When are you doing them at the moment? If you're doing them at the beginning of the day try doing them at the end of the day. Today try varying the time of your First Steps sessions.

The Fat Jar

You should also be managing to weave your Fat Jar Fitness into the fabric of your day: putting your coins in the jar for walking or cycling when you'd have driven in the past, taking the kids to the park and playing football with them, walking up escalators and doing a *Ground Force*-style revamp of the garden.

Challenge: Increasing your Fat Jar Fitness

How about adding some more coins to The Fat Jar today? Find some more ways of taking Fat Burning Pills – what else can you do to put even an extra five pence in the jar?

Feel Good Fitness

I could publish a whole book of the reasons people have given me for giving up on their planned Feel Good Fitness pro-gramme, and I used to try and answer them all individually, until I realised just exactly how unhelpful that was. Nothing works until you work it out for yourself, and the ICB (I Can't Because) exercise is designed to help you do just that.

(DO THIS NOW!)

ICB Syndrome

In your Notebook, draw up two columns, headed like the ones below. Fill in the 'I can't' column first: just write down all the reasons why it's hard for you to do your Feel Good Fitness.

Then, on the other side, write down exactly the same number of reasons why you *can* do it. For example:

I can't because	I can because
I'm too tired	Exercise gives me energy
I work long hours	I'll work more efficiently if I fit in some exercise
The gym closed	I'll work out at home
I'm too busy with the kids	I'll take the kids with me

Challenge: Checking your Feel Good Fitness levels

Have you done your three Feel Good Fitness sessions each week? If not, do what you can today and tomorrow. If you have and you're enjoying them, how about adding in an extra one this week for good measure?

DAY SEVEN

Once again, there are no new exercises, challenges or targets for Day Seven. Just have a great day, and give yourself the chance to digest some of the new material you've been learning this week.

If you're not feeling entirely sure of something, now is a great time to read through again, maybe run through a couple of the exercises, and have a look at your Notebook to see what you've been learning.

Enjoy yourself!

Week Three

WEEK THREE STARTER

FIRST:_____

Have you checked through and compared the past two weeks' Food Profiles? What do they tell you? Think about whether it would be useful for you to continue using the Food Profile or whether it's served its purpose. Have you noticed how you feel when you eat?

How easy are you finding it to keep up with the daily programme? Remember, if you miss a day, just start where you left off and carry straight on again as soon as you can.

Having a blip doesn't mean starting again from the beginning – once you've begun, it's best to carry on. If you get to the end and then feel you didn't quite get all of the ideas, just go through it again, starting at the beginning and working gently through. You'll almost certainly notice things you missed or dismissed first time around.

DO THIS NOW!

Of the techniques I've tried so far, what do I *want* to keep doing, do more of, do better or have another go at?

	Keep doing	Do more of	Do better	Have another go at
First Steps Fitness				
Fat Burning Pills				
Feel Good Fitness				
Filling in the Food Profile				
Using my Notebook to keep track of my progress				
Identifying and getting rid of poor eating habits				
Eating by the Hunger Scale				
Patting myself on the back when I get something right				
Eating without doing anything else at the same time				
Visualising the Future Me				
Experimenting with fruit and vegetables I haven't tried before				
Repeating my Affirmations every day				
Eating less sugar				

Have you noticed where you still need to make some changes?

Once again, you're going to fit in at least three Feel Good Fitness sessions this week. Decide when you're going to be able to make time for them, and write them in both your Notebook and your personal diary right *now* – that way the other pressures of daily life won't be able to squeeze them out. Could you move up to four sessions?

Checklist

You wouldn't drive a car without a basic tool kit, a spare wheel and a reasonable amount of petrol in the tank. In winter you'd take a window scraper and put in anti-freeze. If you want to maintain yourself in the best possible condition, you'll need to carry your own personal survival kit too. I've listed some of these items before, but it's worth thinking about having a daily version and a travel pack as well.

Everyday Survival Kit

- Bottle of water
- Healthy snacks
- Well cushioned trainers so that you can walk comfortably whenever you get the chance
- This book
- Your Notebook and pen

Travel Survival Kit

- All the items on the left-hand side, plus:
- Feel Good Fitness clothes
- Personal Feel Good Fitness kit e.g. resistance bands. There are lots of exercise suggestions in Chapters 5 and 6.

DAY ONE

FIRST: _____

Do you have everything you need to help you succeed with this slimming programme? If not, what's missing? Motivation? Time? Self-esteem? Information? Support? How are you going to get it?

Today's challenges . . .

Motivation

Making positive Visualisation a part of your routine

Think Before You Eat

Eating

Kicking another craving

Exercise

Filling in the Energy Chart

Trying out a new form of Feel Good Fitness

Motivation

How have you been getting on with the Visualisation exercises?

Visualising what you want is a powerful technique and you may well find that it helps you achieve a lot more than simply your slimness goals. See if you can figure out how to attach it to something you do twice a day at least: when you go into the bathroom to clean your teeth perhaps, or out to the garden to water the plants. I'm sure you can find something that would work for you.

Challenge: Making positive Visualisation a part of your routine

Find a way of building the Future You exercise – and any of the others that work particularly well for you – into your daily routine.

And while we're on the subject of visualisation, do you remember me asking you to Define Your Goals on page 42? Right now I want to ask you not *what* you want, but *when and where* you want it. Is there a particular situation that you'd most like to look good in?

- When you're wearing certain clothes?
- Or taking them off?
- A party?
- A wedding?
- A beach?
- A job interview?
- When you're with a certain person you want to impress?

Can you imagine that scene as if you were in it right now, looking slim and wonderful?

Challenge: Think Before You Eat

Remember to keep using Think Before You Eat all week.

Eating

I won't be mentioning keeping up your Food Profile much more from now on as we're introducing some new techniques, but if you want to go on using it, just copy it into your Notebook for as long as you feel you need it.

Cravings

Today we're taking a closer look at what happens when your brain craves food your body doesn't need. Top of the likely list of course is sugar – did you find it easy to live without it for a day? Or did you have any side effects like:

- Headaches?
- Tiredness?
- Lack of concentration?
- Craving something sweet?
- Irritability?

If you answered yes to more than two of those, you may be a bit too dependent on sugar. That's OK – a lot of people are – but if you really want to lose weight, it's going to happen faster if you reduce your sugar intake.

Challenge: Kicking another craving

Think of something other than sugar that you find hard to resist. Write it down in your Notebook now, and see if you can live without it completely for the next twenty-four hours. It doesn't matter what it is – crisps, bacon sandwiches, biscuits, croissants, muffins, chips, coffee – whatever you think you can't live without, live without it for the next twenty-four hours. Once you've lived without it for a day, you can resist the temptation to eat it.

Exercise

We're starting today with a few questions:

- What do I want to achieve with Lighten Up?
- What part does exercise play in achieving it?
- What do I want exercise to do for me?
- What benefits do I get from exercising?
- How does it make me feel?
- What would happen if I didn't exercise at all?
- How can I make my exercise more enjoyable?

The Three Es: Exercise, Eating and Energy

I'd be surprised if you answered those questions without using the word 'energy' at least once. Everybody knows that exercise and eating patterns have something to do with energy levels.

However, the link may not be exactly what we think it is. What do you do when you have a sudden energy dip? Or get stuck in a long, low-energy trough? Most people will either hit the sofa or the carbohydrates – and probably both. Now, that reaction could be a sensible one if you've been for a ten-mile walk or worked all day on a building site, but if you feel worn out at the end (or even in the middle) of a long day at the office, your body may not need either rest or food. You might get a much more satisfactory and sustainable rise in your energy levels from a Feel Good Fitness session, a Fat Burning Pill, or even a First Steps session.

Don't take my word for it, check it out for yourself. Throughout this week I want you to fill in the Energy Chart (see pages 152–153) and find out what effect eating and exercise have on how you feel. Checking your energy levels can tell you a great deal about whether you're eating the right food and taking the right exercise. We've provided an example and a blank Energy Chart, which we'll be asking you to fill in.

Challenge: Filling in the Energy Chart

Make a copy of the Energy Chart in your Notebook for each day of this week. This is definitely one to carry about with you because you are looking for the rises and dips in your energy levels as they relate to what you do and what you eat throughout the day, so that you can take more control over your own life.

Also, if you're just getting into the habit of Feel Good Fitness, it's too early to settle for only one or two activities. Keep trying out new things so you'll have plenty of options.

Challenge: Trying out a new form of Feel Good Fitness

Even if you've already found something you like, there may be even more fun options. Having a wider range of physical activities you enjoy will stop you getting bored and help prevent injury.

	7 a.m.	8 a.m.	9 a.m.	10 a.m.	11 a.m.	12 noon	1 p.m.
High energy level		X 1/2 hour walk to work					X Chicken salad sandwich Fruit
Medium energy level			X Cereal & Coffee	X Working at desk			
Low energy level	X Wake up Coffee & Fruit Juice				X Working at desk	X 1/2 hour jog & stretches	

	7 a.m.	8 a.m.	9 a.m.	10 a.m.	11 a.m.	12 noon	1 p.m.
High energy level							
Medium energy level							
Low energy level							

	2 p.m.	3 p.m.	4 p.m.	5 p.m.	6 p.m.	7 p.m.	8 p.m. onwards	
	X Working at desk							High energy level
		X Walking around office		X Walk home		X Fish, potatoes & veggies Glass wine	X Watch TV	Medium energy level
			X Tea & Fruit		X Pottering around the house			Low energy level

	2 p.m.	3 p.m.	4 p.m.	5 p.m.	6 p.m.	7 p.m.	8 p.m. onwards	
								High energy level
								Medium energy level
								Low energy level

DAY TWO

FIRST:

Run an energy check. How do you feel? Fired up and ready to go? Tired and sluggish? Or somewhere in between? If your energy levels are low, put down the book and do a First Steps session before you read on.

Today's challenges . . .

Motivation

Applying the Before and After Rule

Eating

Killing your Cravings

Exercise

Keeping your exercise levels up

Making your exercise programme work for you

Motivation

The Before and After Rule

*'Before you start anything,
consider how you'll feel when it's over.'*

The Before and After Rule is as universally applicable as Sod's Law and you might think it's just as depressing. It works equally well with decisions about sandwiches and love affairs and, of course, slimming, but you can always ignore it – the pleasure of the moment may be well worth the pain later on.

However, the B & A Rule really comes into it's own when you need motivation to get something done. If you can't get yourself out of bed for your run on a dark winter morning, just spend a couple of minutes thinking how good you'll feel when you get back home again. Imagine how warm and tingling your hands and feet will be, how much you'll enjoy that hot bath and how much better your breakfast will taste when you start feeling hungry. In fact, in any situation where you really want to do something but can't be bothered, just focus on the benefit you'll get afterwards and you'll be up and running (maybe literally) in minutes.

Challenge: Applying the Before and After Rule

Next time your inner critic (or Duck) tells you to sit down and have a cup of tea instead of taking the dog for a brisk walk, apply the B & A Rule. Remind yourself of how much better the tea will taste when you've had ten or fifteen minutes of fresh air and exercise.

Eating

Killing your Cravings

Lighten Up isn't about banning sweets or chips or anything else, but today I'll be showing you how to cope with cravings.

It's easy to get so stuck in the unhealthy eating rut that we never question what we're putting into our bodies, and sometimes we're more conscious of other people's eating habits than our own. Have you ever looked at what other people were buying in the supermarket queue and wondered what they could be thinking of?

When I did the shopping for Lighten Up Workshops my trolley was always full of lard, fruit, vegetables and sweets, and I often used to get comments at the checkout. One day an overweight man in the queue behind me decided to give me a lecture. 'It doesn't matter how much fruit you eat,' he said, 'sooner or later, you're going to put on weight if you're going to eat all that lard. It's not good for you.' The rest of the queue agreed with him.

I looked at his trolley. He had a six-pack of mini pork pies, some bacon, a loaf of white bread, apple turnovers and a bunch of bananas. Apart from the quantity, I couldn't see much difference in the quality, but if I'd pointed that out to him he'd have been pretty indignant.

At the workshops and courses we usually unwrap the lard, mould it into a mini-mountain and invite everyone to stir in their favourite food. The end result, a pile of greasy crisps, chocolate digestives, sausage rolls and sponge cake, has changed the way a lot of people feel about what they eat. You could even try this yourself at home.

(DO THIS NOW!)

Do you like it enough to wear it?

- Point to the bits of you where you'd like to have less fat.

- Now point to the places where fattening foods tend to accumulate if you eat them.

- Think about how that food is going to make you feel after you've eaten it. Is it going to give you energy or drain your energy? Is it going to make you fatter?

- Next time you're triggered to eat for any reason other than hunger, ask yourself 'Do I like this food enough to wear it?'

- Next time you think about eating something that you don't really need, ask yourself, 'How is this going to make me feel, fifteen minutes from now?'

- Finally, add some sound effects to the pictures you're making. 'Yuck' is a good one when you see all that lard wobbling on your thighs. And 'Mmmm' for when you think of fruit and vegetables and all the other Foods To Focus On.

Next time you look at food, pause for a moment and think about whether it's the sort of food you're going to say 'Mmmm' to, or is it going to get a 'Yuck' response?

Now let's take a closer look at the foods you think you'll find it hardest to resist. Nothing is off limits, but I suspect that there's something – or maybe a whole range of things – that have more of a hold on you than you'd like. What about the food you've been trying not to eat over the past few days?

DO THIS NOW!

Conquer Your Cravings

Buy some lard and stir in all your favourite Foods To Limit, mix it all into a mini-mountain and put it in the fridge on a plate. Next time you fancy whatever it is you've chosen as your danger area, go and have a look at the plate in the fridge. Do you really want to put all that sugary, fatty food inside your body?

Challenge: Killing your Cravings

Throughout today, keep a close eye on when – and what – you crave. As soon as you identify a food you have a significant craving for, run it through the Do You Like It Enough To Wear It? routine. Then make your decision about whether to eat it or not.

Exercise

Take a break for a minute and look at yesterday's Energy Chart.

The Energy Chart

What do you notice so far? Is there any correlation between what and when you eat, what you do and how energetic you feel? Like the Food Profile, the Energy chart works best if

- You fill it in as you go along – rather than trying to do it at the end of the day.

- You look for patterns by comparing several charts over a few days – you won't learn much from just one day.

So keep filling it in for the rest of the week and see what you learn from it. Most people are surprised at just how much effect their eating and exercise patterns have on how they feel – and in particular at how much more energy they get from energetic exercise. After a while you'll find it's the days you *don't* exercise that leave you feeling sluggish and debilitated.

Feel Good Fitness Success Factors

I haven't given you much specific advice on Feel Good Fitness because so much depends on what you're doing and how fit you already are, but here are some basic guidelines that will help you keep going for longer.

- **Build up gradually:** if you don't have the time or the strength or the energy to do an hour (or even half an hour) of Feel Good Fitness straight away, that's fine. Get started anyway, and do what you can.

- **Keep your options open:** find several different forms of exercise that you're going to enjoy. If you do different things, you're less likely to get stale, or bored. Of course, if you happen to discover – or re-discover – a sport you love and focus on being competitive, you'll probably want to give that your full attention. If not, try them all.

- **Vary your programme:** this applies not just to your range of Feel Good activities but to the way you do them as well. If you jog, it's fun to go at a different time or try a different route occasionally. If you're weight training ask a personal trainer to advise you about changing your routine, and remember to combine some cardiovascular work for the best results.

- **Make it part of your lifestyle:** you're more likely to keep up your Feel Good Fitness if you make it a part of your social life, or something you do with the family and children. It's easier to keep going, and harder to drop out or miss sessions, if other people are part of the arrangements.

- **Suit yourself:** of course, there's an exception to that rule if the rest of your life is highly social and you rely on your solitary jog or swim in the morning to clear your head for the day. Your Feel Good Fitness works best for you if it fits in with your lifestyle and the kind of person you are.

Challenge: Keeping your exercise levels up

Is today one of your Feel Good Fitness days? If so, make sure you make time for it and think about the Success Factors above to make sure you spend the time doing what's going to work best for you.

If today isn't one of your Feel Good Fitness days, can you fit in more Fat Jar Fitness? Or maybe an extra Feel Good Fitness session even though it's not scheduled?

Challenge: Making your exercise programme work for you

Review where you are with all three levels of the Fat Burning Pyramid and decide whether you could do more.

DAY THREE

FIRST:

Get your Notebook and pen ready today – you'll be writing down some ideas to help you eliminate any persistent eating habits you want finally to get rid of.

Today's challenges . . .

Motivation

Emotional Holes and Habit Holes

Eating

Eating a little bit of something you'd normally eat a lot of

Exercise

Checking your energy levels

Feel Good Fitness

Motivation

You may think that perhaps we're coming at the same problem from a lot of different angles and of course, you're right, we are. But the more problem solving ideas we give you, the better your chances of solving the problem, don't you think?

Let's start today by taking another look at some more ways to fix one of the main reasons for being overweight: eating when we aren't hungry. Most of us do this to fill either an emotional hole or a habit hole.

Emotional Holes

Almost any feeling you don't like can fool you into thinking that food is the solution.

The A–Z of eating when you aren't hungry

Ask yourself, do you ever eat because you're:
[tick as appropriate]

Angry	☐	Jittery	☐	Stressed	☐
Bored	☐	Killing time	☐	Tired	☐
Craving	☐	Lonely	☐	Unhappy	☐
Depressed	☐	Miserable	☐	Victimised	☐
Edgy	☐	Needy	☐	Worried	☐
Frustrated	☐	Overworked	☐	eXasperated	☐
Grumpy	☐	Procrastinating	☐	Yucky	☐
Hurt	☐	Quarrelsome	☐	Zonked	☐
Irritated	☐	Restless	☐		

Filling an emotional hole with food rarely works, but for some people, almost any emotion from depression to elation is a reason for eating. So, if we've got into the habit of reaching for the fudge cake when we're feeling down (or when we're feeling up and we want to celebrate), it's because we have learned that eating is an easy, quick-fix response in lots of situations.

DO THIS NOW!

Write down a non-hunger need that you generally fill with food and then write down some alternative, low-calorie ways to meet it instead. For example, if you often find yourself eating cheesecake in front of the TV because you're lonely, you could go for a walk, do some ironing, phone a friend, brush the cat or water the plants.

The emotional hole I'm most likely to fill with food is

_____

I could meet that need by

1. _____
2. _____
3. _____
4. _____
5. _____

Habit Holes

The second reason for ignoring the Hunger Scale is even easier to deal with – it's simply habit. There doesn't have to be an underlying reason, like eating to keep yourself awake at the computer or comforting yourself with chocolate when you're lonely. You might have popcorn at the cinema just because everybody else does, or snack when you get in from work because you always used to eat straight after school.

Over the past couple of weeks I've been suggesting you make a note of all the habits and triggers that make you eat when you aren't hungry. You probably have your own list by now – how many of them have you managed to eliminate?

It's easier to get rid of habits if you remember that they live in the holes in your life. If you want to get rid of one permanently, you need to fill the hole immediately. Otherwise the habit will creep right back in again.

(DO THIS NOW!)

Write down the eating habit you want to break. Then think of ways you could fill that habit hole without eating.

Eating habit: _____

Instead of eating I could fill that habit hole with

1. _____
2. _____
3. _____
4. _____
5. _____

Eating for the wrong reasons

I've said it before, but it won't hurt to say it again – eating when you're registering less than six or seven on the Hunger Scale will make you put on weight. The end result will be the same whether you're eating out of habit or emotional need, but it's easier to tackle the causes if we look at them separately.

Challenge: Emotional Holes and Habit Holes

Do the two exercises above and then, if you have some more habits you still need to deal with, just write them in your Notebook and list some alternatives to eating underneath each one.

Eating

So far today we've been looking at how you can spend less time eating when you aren't hungry. Now let's take a look at how you can spend more time eating when you *are* hungry.

It's not about eating more food, it's about taking more time over it so that you

- Enjoy it more.

- Get a better feel for what really tastes good and what doesn't.

- Know when you're full in time to stop.

I know I've already talked about eating more slowly and I wonder how you're getting on with that?

How many of these have you done in the last week?

- Putting your knife and fork down between mouthfuls.

- Taking the serving dishes off the table when everyone has had a helping – even if there's food left in them.

- Eating without doing anything else.

- Pausing between courses.

Challenge: Eating a little bit of something you'd normally eat a lot of

Buy your favourite snack bar, packet of crisps or sweets and sit down with it. Take it bite by bite, asking yourself how it really tastes and how it's making you feel. Halfway through it, stop for five minutes, get up and do something else. Then ask yourself, 'do I still want to finish it?' If you do, then go ahead, but take your time, make it last and think about what it is that makes it taste so good.

Exercise

Unless you already have a physically exhausting job, you'll probably find that exercise will give you energy rather than taking it away.

Challenge: Checking your energy levels

Pay attention to the effect that activity has on your energy levels and mark it on your Energy Chart, making a note of the results.

	More tired	No change	More energy
Feel Good Fitness			
Fat Jar Fitness			
First Steps Fitness			
Sitting down for more than an hour			

Challenge: Feel Good Fitness

If today's one of your three (or preferably four) Feel Good Fitness days, make sure you make time for it.
If it's not, make sure you're as active as you can be.

DAY FOUR

FIRST: _____

Check your Goal Statement. Has it changed? If so write it down again – you'll be needing it in a minute.

Today's challenges . . .

Motivation

Eliminating negative beliefs

Eating

Food without labels

Exercise

Varying your exercise routine

Coordinating your body and brain

Motivation

Belief Building

Remember the Slimming Scale on page 100 and the lists of negative and positive words you made? Did you turn the positive words into Affirmations and build them into positive new beliefs?

If you did that exercise again now, do you think you'd pick the same words? What would you like to believe about your size and shape, your fitness and health today? If you come up with anything new, write it in your Notebook now.

Affirmation is just one of the tools you can use to help strengthen your new beliefs about yourself as a slim, fit and healthy person. Today we'll be looking at some other ways of reinforcing those positive beliefs.

(DO THIS NOW!)

What Makes You Think You're Winning?

Make a list in your Notebook of all the things that support your belief in the progress you're making. Are you taking more exercise? Drinking more water? Eating healthier food?

- _____
- _____
- _____
- _____

Imagine one of your positive beliefs – 'I'm getting slimmer, fitter and healthier' perhaps – written in huge letters on the top of a table. Spray-painting your belief on to a tabletop is a great start, but the tabletop isn't going to stand up without legs – and the table legs are all the positive things you are doing to support the belief.

DO THIS NOW!

Write down your Goal Statement
e.g. 'I want to be slimmer'

Turn it into an affirmation
e.g. 'I am getting slimmer'

Believe in your affirmation

Carve the belief into your imaginary table top

Build the legs to make it stand up

'I'm doing my First Steps exercises every day'
'I'm fitting four or more Fat Jar breaks into every day'
'I'm starting a Feel Good Fitness programme'
'I'm drinking at least two litres of water a day'
'I'm eating more fruit and vegetables'
'I'm feeling good about myself'
'I've succeeded in other things, I can succeed in slimming too'

What other legs can you add to support the positive belief?

_____

_____

_____

_____

Zapping the beliefs you don't want

You can get rid of negative beliefs very simply by reversing this process. If you remove the foundations, it's going to be impossible to believe negative things about yourself. For instance:

- If you believe you're always going to be overweight and underactive, just hack away at the table legs supporting that belief. Start eating fruit instead of chocolate biscuits, go for a walk instead of watching TV, and picture yourself looking wonderful all the time.

- If you believe you'll never enjoy exercise, try lots of different activities until you find one that's fun for you.

- If you believe you'll never enjoy Food To Focus On, experiment with more exciting recipes and foods you haven't tried before.

Challenge: Eliminating negative beliefs

Eliminate a negative belief that you still have about yourself.

Eating

Goodies and Baddies and the rest

I've already talked about sugar and fat because they are both pretty scary to dedicated dieters. I've also mentioned fruit and vegetables because we all know they're good for us, although we still don't eat enough of them. I've mentioned water, too, because although it's sensible (and fashionable) to carry a bottle around with you, people still seem to prefer tea, coffee and soft drinks.

However, there are some other food groups that are extremely important to our well being, like protein for example, and essential fatty acids. For more details have a look at Chapter 7.

If you still feel confused sometimes about what you need to eat and what you don't, make a copy of the Food Profile and stick it on the fridge just as a reminder of what to focus on.

Life's too short to read labels

We always used to tell people to read the labels on packaged food and check what was in it, but life's too short to read lots of labels. If a fruit yoghurt has a long label then it's obviously got too many ingredients – how much space does it take to write *'yoghurt, fruit & sugar'*? Most of the extra ingredients will have no nutritional value – and what's the point of putting something inside you if you can't taste it and it has no nutritional value? Buy a plain yoghurt instead – you can make the decision about whether it's high fat or low fat – and add your own fruit. Add your own sugar as well if you must – at least you'll know how much of it you're eating.

Challenge: Food without labels

See if you can get through a whole day on food that doesn't have labels.

Exercise

The Fat Burning Pyramid

Has your Fat Burning Pyramid turned into a solid structure yet – or are you still working on it? Today I'm going to suggest you vary it just a little bit.

It's easy for a routine to become a rut – especially with exercise. You may be thinking, 'It's hard enough to fit in all those First Steps sessions and all that brisk exercise in the first place – and now I've got to change it?' But I'm not suggesting anything drastic, just that you look at when and how you're doing it now, and change the balance a bit. For example, if most of your activity's been in the evening up to now, see if you can fit some into the morning somewhere. You'll find it very interesting to check the effect on your Energy Chart when you exercise at the very beginning and very end of the day.

> ## Challenge: Varying your exercise routine
>
> Make a deliberate change to the timing or order of your Fat Jar breaks and Feel Good Fitness today and see what effect that has on your energy. Perhaps you could leave work on time and do some exercise in the evening, rather than getting up earlier in the morning, or go for a brisk walk at lunchtime?

You'll also find the exercise you do much more productive if you engage your brain as well as your body.

You will get so much more benefit from workouts where you focus your mind on what your body is doing. Exercising with your mind on your body is a physical form of meditation. If you want a better body, give the one you've got the attention it deserves. When you're doing resistance training, for example, pay attention to the muscle groups you're working. Imagine the energy you're generating, imagine the power you're getting, imagine those muscles the way you want them to be.

Why? Because you get what you focus on. So focus on what you want.

Challenge: Coordinating your body and your brain

Body warm-up:
Remember to take an extra minute or two for a warm-up session before you do your Feel Good Fitness, and make time for a cool-down afterwards (you could even use the First Steps routine for this, or the stretching exercises in Chapter 6).

Brain Warm-up:
You'll get more benefit from any exercise you do if you get your brain tuned into it first. Just check the answers to these questions before you start a Feel Good Fitness session. You could also do it before you take a Fat Burning Pill.

- How will this exercise make me feel if I do it?

- How will it make me feel if I don't do it?

- How will it make me feel two hours from now?

- How will it make me feel this time tomorrow?

You're a dream team, not just a body carrying around a brain. It's always a good idea to check with your brain before activating your body, and it's also a good idea to run a reality check with your body before your brain makes a decision.

DAY FIVE

FIRST:

- *What's your energy level right now? Are you fired up and ready to go? Relaxed? Tired? Edgy?*

- *What is it that's put you in that state? Eating? Exercise? Too much sleep? Too little sleep?*

- *If you aren't happy with the way you feel right now, what can you do to fix it before you read on?*

Today's challenges . . .

Motivation

Using the B & A Rule

Rewarding yourself

Eating

Noticing how your eating patterns affect your energy levels

Exercise

Taking a Feel Good Fitness break without
any other distractions

Motivation

The Before and After Rule

There does seem to be a basic human instinct to hang on to good experiences as if they'll never come around again. Eating can be a truly wonderful experience – but it's much much more pleasurable when we're truly hungry. When we eat beyond hunger, it's not so intense – but we still do it. Remember the Before and After Rule? It says: 'Before you start anything, consider how you'll feel when it's over.' In other words: don't do anything unless it's going to feel just as good afterwards as it did while you were doing it!

There is no downside to thoroughly enjoying your food *if* you are hungry. So stop punishing yourself when you get things wrong and start congratulating yourself when you get things right. Give yourself some positive feedback when you use a Lighten Up technique successfully and reinforce those good habits you're developing.

Challenge: Using the Before and After Rule

Make sure you use the B & A Rule every time you eat today.

Challenge: Rewarding yourself

Think of a new way to reward yourself when you notice positive changes. If you're eating when you're hungry, stopping when you're full, and fitting in your Fat Jar Fitness, buy yourself a treat that has nothing to do with food – a trip to the cinema, a CD, time out to do something you want, or maybe a massage.

Eating

The Energy Chart

The Energy Chart is usually in the Exercise section of the daily programme, but today I've moved it into the Eating section because I want you to notice the effect on your energy levels of what you eat as well as what you do.

Eating and Energy

Food and Drink	Hunger Scale Reading	More tired	No change	More energy

---

Challenge: Noticing how your eating patterns affect your energy levels

Notice how your eating patterns affect your energy levels today and write them all down in your Notebook.

Exercise

Back on page 103 we talked about eating without distractions – it's an idea you can also apply to exercise. If you watch someone take that first sip from a glass of wine, or the first nibble from a bar of chocolate, they often close their eyes and concentrate on the pleasure of the moment. Your brain is releasing similar chemicals when you exercise – so why aren't you paying attention?

Challenge: Taking a Feel Good Fitness break without any other distractions

If you have a Feel Good Fitness session today, see if you can do it without any distractions.

If today isn't one of your three (or four) Feel Good Fitness days this week, then make sure you really concentrate on all your First Steps exercises and Fat Jar breaks.

DAY SIX

FIRST: _____

Look through your Notebook and see if you've made a note of times in the last three weeks when you've lapsed, overeaten or missed your exercise. Can you remember how it happened and what you did about it?

Today's challenges . . .

Motivation

Setting Outcomes that will lead you to your slimming goal

Eating

Cutting down on Foods To Limit

Exercise

Focusing on your body

Using exercise to break out of an eating lapse

Motivation

I've been giving you some regular reminders about re-visiting and updating your goals. One way of making goals more achievable is to build Stepping-stones so that you can take one small, safe step at a time.

Outcomes

If you call these Stepping-stones Outcomes, you can set some useful, achievable ones every day that will take you closer to your goal. For example, you might say to yourself: 'This morning I'll take a Fat Burning Pill twice and have salad instead of a burger for lunch.' Right there you have three Outcomes or Stepping-stones before you're even halfway through your day.

The great thing about Outcomes is that the ones you do achieve are still valid, even if you don't manage them all. The two Fat Burning Pills are taking you nearer your goal, for example, even if you have the burger instead of the salad for lunch.

Lapse, Relapse, Collapse

You know what I mean by lapsing, relapsing and collapsing – somebody offers you a cake in the morning because it's their birthday. You accept and decide, as you've now gone off your diet, that you'll have fish and chips and a pudding for lunch.

However, once you start to think in terms of Outcomes, it takes the terror out of the old lapse, relapse, collapse routine. When you realise a cake is a self-contained event, and doesn't invalidate your walking to work and doing your First Steps sessions when you got there, you've broken the power of the collapse pattern.

So, to clarify:

- A Lapse is a slight error or slip, a little backslide. It's not the end of the world, and it doesn't mean you have to have a relapse.

- A Relapse is stringing together a whole series of lapses.

- Collapse happens when you start believing your old negative beliefs. Given the tools and techniques you now have at your fingertips, and given the changes you've already made, this is a very unlikely scenario.

Challenge: Setting Outcomes that will lead you to your slimming goal

Set yourself three Outcomes for today. Write them in your Notebook and have a look at them again at the end of the day. Remember, they're all important steps towards your long-term goal.

Eating

Five a Day

On page 172 I asked you to eat food without labels for a whole day – most people find they eat more fruit and vegetables when they do this. What did you do? What effect did it have on you?

On page 177 I asked you to make a special note on your Energy Chart about what you ate. Did your change of eating pattern make any difference, compared to the way your Chart was looking during the first part of this week?

Staying slim means eating more healthy food, but I know you won't actually do it unless you experience for yourself how much better it makes you feel. So ask yourself:

What is it about eating and drinking that makes a difference to the way I feel?

- Is it the time of day?
- Is it how much I eat?
- Is it the kind of food I eat?
- Fat?

- Sugar?
- Carbohydrates?
- Stimulants?
- What else?

Did you see any other patterns from the Energy Chart over the past week?

_____

_____

_____

Challenge: Cutting down on Foods To Limit

Eat as few Foods To Limit as possible today. Think about how this makes you feel. Make sure you eat the kind of food that keeps your energy levels high and steady – your aim is to feel good all day.

Exercise

Focusing on you

Did you go for a Feel Good Fitness session yesterday, and did you really focus on what you were doing, rather than distracting yourself? If you did, how did it feel?

Challenge: Focusing on your body

Today, whenever you do some Feel Good or Fat Jar exercise, or when you do one of your First Steps sessions, focus totally on your body and the muscles you're using and be aware, all the time, of your breathing.

Exercise Wheel review

Take a minute and fill the Exercise Wheel in again. Have your activity patterns changed in the last three weeks? If not, what else can you do to get more movement into your daily life?

Challenge: Using exercise to break out of an eating lapse

Next time you have a lapse with your healthy eating plan, see if you can use either a First Steps session or a Fat Burning Pill to break the pattern.

DAY SEVEN

Of course, once again there are no new exercises, challenges or targets for Day Seven. As in Weeks One and Two, Day Seven is for you to take the time to sit back, relax and mentally consolidate everything you've been learning.

And to prepare yourself for the final week!

Week Four

WEEK FOUR STARTER

FIRST: _____

*Where are you on the Motivation Scale and the Feel Good Scale?
Are you nearer ten than one? Are you scoring higher than you did
back in Chapters 2 and 3? Changing your negative beliefs to positive
ones (Chapter 4) will help you feel more optimistic and confident
of success.*

Before you move on to the next week's challenges, give yourself
a better chance of succeeding by checking where you are on the
Feel Good Scale. If you aren't as high, or higher, than last time,
maybe some Feel Good Fitness, a Fat Burning Pill or even a
First Steps session would boost your levels of happy chemicals:
the Fat Burning Pyramid can be a good place to visit when
you're feeling down.

You can use the following list to check your progress.

DO THIS NOW!

Of the techniques you learned, what do you *want* to keep doing, do more of, try again or leave for now? If there are any that I haven't mentioned, just add them to the end of the list.

Mark them all according to how well they've worked for you:

- 3 stars against the ones you're using daily.
- 2 stars against the ones you're using fairly regularly.
- 1 star against the ones you tried only once.
- leave a blank against the ones you haven't done yet.

	★	★★	★★★
First Steps Fitness			
Fat Jar breaks			
Feel Good Fitness			
Using my Notebook to keep track of my progress			
Substituting new, good habits for old, negative ones			
Eating by the Hunger Scale			
Finding ways to reward myself when I do well			
Meeting my emotional holes directly instead of filling them with food			
Building new positive beliefs that support me in becoming slimmer, fitter and healthier			

⇨

	★	★★	★★★
Slowing down my eating			
Seeing the Future Me			
Filling in the gaps in my Foods To Focus On – especially eating more fruit and vegetables			
Eating complex carbohydrates instead of sugar			
Drinking plenty of water			
Using the Success Formula			
Monitoring my energy levels according to what I eat and what I do			
Changing my relationship with the foods I crave the most			

This will tell you a lot about how much effort you're really putting into this. The more triple stars you have, the sooner you'll see changes.

Check your Motivation Scale. The chances are that filling in this list will have pushed up your score, and motivation is a major success factor.

Exercise

You're now moving into the last phase of the four-week plan, and it's really worth going for it this week! You should have been doing three (or maybe even four) Feel Good Fitness sessions per week for the last fortnight. This week decide which days you can fit your sessions in, and write them in your Notebook and your diary.

Remember to keep going with your First Steps sessions and Fat Jar Fitness as well.

Checklist

There's just one item on the list – a new Notebook. Except that this time it won't just be a Notebook, this time it's a Diary you'll be needing, or at least something you can lay out in date order. You'll be using it in Chapter 4 to keep track of your new Lighten Up For Life programme, but you can start straight away if you like.

The Diary will be your Slimming Buddy for the rest of your life – or for as long as you need it. If you use it for just a couple of minutes a day to note down what went right and what didn't, it will show you the patterns in your life. It will help you keep track of what helped you change.

DAY ONE

FIRST:

Check where you are on the Motivation Scale.

Today's challenges . . .

Motivation

Combining your Affirmations with your First Steps exercises

Writing your own Success Formula

Eating

Following the Food Profile Programme

Eliminating any remaining poor habits

Exercise

Making Feel Good Fitness a part of your everyday life

Motivation

Lighten Up is about freeing yourself from all the limiting beliefs and habits of the past by learning to rely on your own resources rather than depending on diets.

The Awareness Habit

Knowing where you are in terms of motivation and feeling good about yourself is very important. It's easy to start slimming on a wave of enthusiasm (or disgust) and in the first few weeks, when things are going well, you don't notice your old habits and feelings gradually creeping up on you again.

Keeping a check on your emotions means you'll see when you're sliding towards the vulnerable end of any of the scales. Then you can take control again with one of the Lighten Up techniques: looking back over your own achievements, visualising the Future You, saying your Affirmations or stepping right out of your physical space and doing a First Steps session or taking a Fat Burning Pill.

You could even try combining a couple of different Lighten Up techniques next time you notice your confidence taking a dip, and that's the first challenge for today:

Challenge: Combining your Affirmations with your First Steps exercises

Make up a new Affirmation for yourself today and repeat it every time you do your First Steps programme.

The Success Formula

The Success Formula is a great way to deal with the challenges people often face and sets you up for a successful outcome. It's incredibly simple – the only catch is you actually have to do it!

DO THIS NOW!

The Success Formula

Think of a time when you had a lapse, then you strung together a whole series of lapses and binged for a day or didn't exercise. Now re-live that experience, step by step, looking at it from a different point of view:

Step One
Remember what happened – the first slip that triggered the landslide: the first crisp that made you eat the whole packet; the first morning you stayed in bed instead of exercising and it felt so good you took the whole week off.

Identify the point where you could still say 'Ah ha! I know what's happening to me now – and I know how it usually ends – but I'm still strong enough at this moment to *do something different.*'

Step Two
STOP. Interrupt that memory for a moment. What exactly was going on?

Step Three
Imagine you're actually talking to yourself at the time it's happening – but you aren't giving yourself a hard time, you're just asking yourself what on earth you think you're doing. Be curious about what made you behave the way you did. Laugh at it. The behaviour isn't important. Your response to it is what matters.

Ask yourself some useful questions:

- 'What triggered me to do that?'
- 'How did I lose control?'
- 'What was in my mind just before I did it?'
- 'What made me so vulnerable just then?'

Step Four

When you understand why you did what you did, ask yourself:

'What will I do differently next time it happens, so that I get a different result – one that doesn't make me feel so bad about myself?'

Think about all the possible alternative courses of action you could have taken at the time:

- going for a walk
- phoning a friend
- having a bath

Challenge: Writing your own Success Formula

You've really already done this by doing the exercise above, but now convert it to a strategy and write it in your Notebook. We tend to repeat our mistakes so, sooner or later, that strategy is bound to come in very handy.

Eating

Remember that *you* can control how you feel about food. If food has had a hold on you in the past and you really want to break free from it, the power is in your hands.

Challenge: Following the Food Profile Programme

Select at least one thing from each section of the Foods To Focus On circle. Try something different. And why not try some new recipes from Chapter 8?

Challenge: Eliminating any remaining poor habits

Write down and eliminate any poor habits you're still holding on to.

Exercise

(**DO THIS NOW!**)

How could you make Feel Good Fitness and Fat Jar Fitness an essential part of your leisure time activities?

- What are your five favourite leisure pursuits?
  1. _____
  2. _____
  3. _____
  4. _____
  5. _____

- How many of them involve physical activity?

- Could you substitute active leisure activities for some of the sedentary ones you listed? What would they be?
  1. _____
  2. _____
  3. _____
  4. _____
  5. _____

- Would any of the rest of your family and friends be interested in joining you?

- Could you take up something that would involve the kids – like swimming or cycling?

- Do any of your family and friends already have active leisure interests that you could join in?

- Could you adapt anything you already do to make it a bit more energetic – pulling your own golf trolley perhaps instead of driving round in an electric cart, or even walking out to a restaurant rather than going by car?

Challenge: Making Feel Good Fitness a part of your everyday life

If today is one of your four days for Feel Good Fitness, try out a new activity.

If it isn't, make sure you know when your next Feel Good Fitness days are and really think about making Feel Good Fitness an essential part of your life.

DAY TWO

FIRST:

Decide on some Outcomes/Stepping-stones to be your goal for today and write them in your Diary.

Today's challenges . . .

Motivation

The Movie

Eating

Drinking only water (while eating normally) for the next twenty-four hours

Exercise

Outcomes

Motivation

Visualisation is one of the most powerful and creative ways of using your mind to help you achieve your goals. Some people find it easier than others to do it straight away, but in the end it works for everybody who's prepared to do it regularly.

Today we're taking Visualisation a step further and turning it into a movie.

(DO THIS NOW!)

The Movie

Like all Visualisation exercises, it's often easier if you have someone talking you through it for the first couple of times at least. You can even do it over the phone with your Slimming Buddy if you can't get together. It's also perfect for listening to on a tape and you could record your own voice if you wanted to do that.

- Imagine you're looking at a glossy magazine. It's open at a double-page spread of the film that has just been made about your life. The pictures in the article show some of your greatest moments. There you are, looking slim, fit and healthy as you achieve your personal goals, your career goals and your slimming goals as well.

- Pick three of your favourite photos from the magazine article and spread them out in front of you. Have a good look at them and congratulate yourself – you did well and you look wonderful.

- You're going to turn those three photos into a five-minute video of highlights from the film, directed by you. So sit in your imaginary Director's Chair and take the first image, the one of you looking so slim and successful, and project it on to the huge screen in front of you. ⇨

- Take a good look at that image and then project the second and third images on to the screen, one at a time. Finally put them all up on the screen together, in whatever order makes sense to you.

- Look at the three photos and notice what it is that makes them so compelling and attractive.

- Now, run together as a film the three experiences that those photos come from. They may be totally different, but that's fine. Turn them into a colourful action movie with your favourite music as the soundtrack. Watch it right through a couple of times from beginning to end.

- Rewind to the beginning and, as the first frame comes up on the screen again, step into it. As you step into it, repeat your Affirmation – the one you were saying to yourself yesterday while you were doing your First Steps programme.

- Stay in the movie from start to finish, starring in your own life. Imagine yourself doing whatever you were doing in the three original photographs: meeting your challenges, playing with your children, running on the beach, walking into your new job or having fun with your friends.

- You're looking at the film set through your own eyes, seeing and hearing everything as it happens. What are you feeling? Are you happy? Ecstatic? Overwhelmed? Tearful?

- When you've lived through those scenes, step down from the screen and sit back in your Director's Chair again. Take a deep breath and relax. Now that you've experienced it from the inside, play it through again once more while you watch and ask yourself how you would describe that star you are watching on the screen:

  o She really worked for that – she deserves it.

  o He looks like he knows how to have fun.

○ She's got her priorities right.

○ He's got staying power and determination.

○ She's looking good – she obviously takes care of herself.

○ He looks so happy and healthy.

You can run endless variations on this – adding to the experiences as you go through life.

Challenge: The Movie

Take time out to run the Movie in your mind three or four times today. Get used to the idea of being a star.

Eating

The Last Word On Diets

We used to spend a lot of time talking about why dieting makes it hard to stay slim, until we realised that by the time people turn to Lighten Up they already know diets don't work.

Some of the most popular diets are also the most difficult to follow – either because they are anti-social or because they run contrary to our normal eating instincts and weight loss happens mainly because it's difficult to eat as much as you normally would. You're unlikely to stick with them for long – which is just as well because living by such rigid rules may put you at risk of missing out on some vital nutrients, as well as keeping you completely out of touch with how hungry you are and what your body needs.

So, are you ready to do things differently? Are you ready to give up:

- the sharp, short-term weight loss

- and the overall, long-term steady weight gain?

If you take the decision to live without those dieting certainties you've come to depend on and go for Lighten Up instead, what are we offering you in return?

- A healthy, balanced eating plan that is specifically tailored by you to meet your body's needs.

- A more active lifestyle which will turn your body into a fat burning machine and give you a great deal of pleasure and satisfaction.

- A positive, powerful way of thinking which will make it easy for you to stay slim, fit and healthy for life – and probably a lot happier as well.

Challenge: Drinking only water (while eating normally) for the next twenty-four hours

Just for today, eliminate soft drinks, tea, coffee and alcohol.
Make sure you fit in at least two litres of water, making a note
of how you feel.

Exercise

A Slimmer Lifestyle

The First Steps sessions, Fat Jar Fitness and Feel Good Fitness will make you slimmer if you weave them into the fabric of your life.

On page 180 we talked about setting yourself daily Outcomes which would act as Stepping-stones to your goal. Well, building a Fat Burning Pyramid is an Outcome in itself. If you fit the Fat Burning Pyramid into your daily life, your route to health and fitness will be so solid that you'll never even think about your weight again. Staying slim will become something you'll take for granted.

(DO THIS NOW!)

**Here are some ready-made Exercise Outcomes
– pick one from each level and make it
your own for today**

Fat Building Pyramid	I'm going to build a whole Fat Burning Pyramid today.
Feel Good Fitness	My outcome for my Feel Good Fitness session today is to: • Feel energised at the end of it. • Vary my weights routine. • Try a new exercise.
Fat Jar Fitness	My outcome for my Fat Jar Fitness sessions today is to: • Make sure they are evenly spread through the day.

⇨

- Do two of my sessions in the evening, before and after dinner.

- Split my sessions up into an hourly five-minute break instead of just three fifteen minute chunks.

First Steps Fitness

My outcome for my First Steps exercises today is to:

- Do at least three of them out of doors.

- Do them to some music I enjoy.

- Do a First Steps session every time I check the Hunger Scale.

Challenge: Outcomes

Pick an Outcome from each category in the list above, write it in your Notebook, and make sure you achieve it today. For example:

- I'm going to try a new Feel Good Fitness activity today.

- I'm going to spread my Fat Jar Fitness sessions evenly throughout the day today.

- I'm going to do a First Steps session every time I check the Hunger Scale today.

DAY THREE

FIRST:_____

Check the Outcomes you set for yourself yesterday – did you achieve them?

Today's challenges . . .

Motivation

Planning your future

Eating

Eliminating poor eating habits

Exercise

Eliminating poor exercise habits

Motivation

The Good Habit Guide

There's one word that crops up in this book almost as often as slimming (and a lot more often than calories or weight). The key word is 'habits' – and you already know that the best way to get rid of poor habits permanently is to install new, good ones.

We live a lot of our daily lives according to habit. If we didn't we'd have to make decisions about every tiny little thing we do and life would get very tiring. So, building up a solid framework of good eating and exercise habits that will support us in achieving our goals is a really good idea.

A lot of things you do might not look like habits first time around. You might even think those habits make you who you are. Don't be fooled – especially in the areas of eating and exercise. Habits are just habits and you can decide whether you change them or keep them.

It's not part of you – it's just something you do

Simply re-labelling your overeating, under-exercising and negative thinking as mere poor habits, takes away their power to control your life. It puts you in charge again. You can *choose* not to overeat or watch too much TV or feel bad about yourself. You can even *choose* to eat more Food To Focus On, be more active and start believing the positive Affirmations you've stuck all over your kitchen.

Why do some people find that overeating and under-exercising are such difficult habits to break?

- Because you can't give up food completely.

- Because the less you exercise, the less fit you may be and the more difficult and uncomfortable exercise will become.

- Because dieting, the most popular method of weight management, tends to focus on food making your cravings even worse.

The good news

The good news is that, slowly and surely, all the ideas and techniques I've described in this book will help you to get back the healthy eating and exercise habits you were born with.

Challenge: Planning your future

In your Notebook and new Diary make a list of five things you still want to do – things you've dreamed of but never done before. Imagine the Future You, looking slim, fit and healthy, doing all of those things.

_____

_____

_____

_____

Eating

While we're on the subject of habits, let's take a look at how you got on with changing your drinking habits over the last twenty-four hours. How do you feel after twenty-four hours of drinking just water? Would you want to do it again occasionally? If so, why?

- Because it made you feel good?

- Because it made you realise how little water you usually drink?

- Because it helped you realise you might have under-estimated your tea, coffee and soft drink consumption when you filled in the Food Profile?

We are often even less aware of how much or how little we drink than of how much we eat. Since so many of us don't drink enough water (we need about two litres a day) it's something you may want to think about.

DO THIS NOW!

Eating & Drinking Habits to Develop	Eating & Drinking Habits to Ditch
Tick the ones you already do and want to develop – and give yourself a pat on the back.	*Cross out any of the ones I've put in that don't apply to you, and add your personal list of unhelpful eating habits.*
Drinking at least two litres of water a day.	Drinking more alcohol, tea, coffee and soft drinks than plain water.
Eating at least five portions of fruit and vegetables a day.	Continuing to eat when you're full.

Eating & Drinking Habits to Develop

Eating a rainbow – getting a good range of colours on your plate.

Eating as many fresh, unprocessed foods as possible.

Eating foods from all the segments of the Foods To Focus On Circle.

Putting your knife and fork down between mouthfuls.

Eating without doing anything else at the same time.

Eating when you're at six or seven on the Hunger Scale.

Pausing between courses to give your stomach time to register if it's full.

Always having healthy foods at hand in case you get hungry and you aren't at home.

Eating & Drinking Habits to Ditch

Eating more from the Foods To Limit Circle than Foods To Focus On – fill in the ones you find it hardest to resist:

_____

_____

_____

Eating when you aren't hungry (fill in your own reasons):

_____

_____

_____

Fill in any more unhelpful eating habits:

_____

_____

_____

_____

Challenge: Eliminating poor eating habits

When you've checked through both lists, make a note in your future Diary of how you plan to ditch the habits on the right.

Exercise

The Fat Burning Pyramid

The Fat Burning Pyramid is a solid structure of good exercise habits that you can build into your lifestyle. It will support you through your motivational down days so you won't have to say to yourself, 'Will I squeeze in my First Steps exercises today? Or will I have to skip them?' The layers of the pyramid will be part of your life so that it takes a very drastic change of routine indeed to knock you off course.

Although you will get temporarily side-tracked occasionally – there will be days when there's an emergency, or you aren't well, or you have to travel – that's fine, because the structure will be built in by then, so you know you can always come back to it.

DO THIS NOW!

Exercise Habits

Exercise Habits to Develop	Exercise Habits to Ditch
Just like you did with the eating and drinking habits, tick the ones you already do and want to develop. Don't forget to congratulate yourself.	*Delete the ones you don't do and add any of your own that I didn't mention.*
First Steps Fitness: Fitting your First Steps exercises into your day is a great habit to have.	Missing your Feel Good Fitness session because you've had a stressful day. Exercise is a great relaxer and energiser.
Fat Jar Fitness: Fitting in four or more is a brilliant habit to have. You will probably find that you stop counting Fat Burning Pills as you get more and more into the habit of leading an active life.	Using the car for short journeys, because you can't leave the kids, carry the shopping or maybe because it's raining.

Exercise Habits to Develop

Feel Good Fitness: It may take a little longer to make a habit out of this – First Steps Fitness and Fat Jar Fitness are easier to weave into the pattern of your life. But if you can make Feel Good Fitness a part of your daily routine as well, you'll find yourself doing it without a second thought.

Paying attention to signals from your body: If you're physically more tired than usual you could be unwell, so have a night off or take it easy. Never exercise when you're injured.

Pacing yourself and using the Borg Scale to make sure you stay within safe, motivational, useful limits.

Exercise Habits to Ditch

Exercising infrequently. For Feel Good Fitness, twice a week is the absolute minimum and three sessions are better. If you exercise infrequently you run the risk of injury or demotivation.

Being in such a hurry to get your Feel Good Fitness over and done with that you don't do a proper warm-up and cool-down.

Over-exercising – it's tempting, if you don't get to the gym or the squash court very often, to go flat out for as long as you can.

Fill in the exercise habits you want to ditch:

_____

_____

_____

Challenge: Eliminating poor exercise habits

Write your plan for emptying the list on the right in your future Diary.

DAY FOUR

FIRST:

Where are you, right now, on the Feel Good Scale? Stop for a moment and run your Movie in your mind. Now check the Feel Good Scale again. What's the difference?

Today's challenges . . .

Motivation

Being your own best friend

Setting up your own Feel Good Factory

Eating

Enjoying your food

Foods To Focus On

Exercise

The Borg Scale

Motivation

'This week's homework is to get to know yourself better and start being nice to yourself,' I said.

Jane's hand went up. 'The reason I'm here is because I've spent too many years being nice to myself and I've finally realised I've got to start being tougher.'

'How may times have you tried being tough on yourself?'

'Every time I've been on a diet I suppose.'

'Did it work?'

'No.'

The only way you'll ever adopt a lifestyle that includes the Hunger Scale, Think Before You Eat and the Fat Burning Pyramid is by believing that you are truly worth it. So, here's your homework for the rest of the week:

- Continue getting to know yourself better so that you can meet your body's real needs.

- Find ways other than food or inertia to comfort, reward and energise yourself.

DO THIS NOW!

Ask yourself:

- What sort of thing do I say when I talk to myself?
- Do I treat myself as well as I treat my best friend?
- If not, what do I do differently?
- What sort of messages do I give myself?
- For example?

_____

_____

- What do I talk to my friends about?

- What do I read?

- The majority of television programmes, especially the soaps, focus on disasters and dysfunctional behaviours. What do I watch?

- Where is my attention – on solutions or problems?

When you've answered these questions to your own satisfaction you'll have a better idea of why you feel as good – or as bad – as you do most of the time.

Remember:

- Depriving yourself of food when you're hungry or eliminating certain types of food from your diet is not treating yourself well – and neither is going to the gym twice a week and working yourself past ten on the Borg Scale, and then sitting down for the rest of the week.

- Stuffing yourself with too much of the wrong kind of food and ignoring your body's need for maintenance is not treating yourself well. Giving yourself sweets when you really want time and attention is not even treating yourself like an adult.

Challenge: Being your own best friend

Be your own best friend for the rest of the week. Then, if you're getting on well, you could think about doing it for the rest of your life.

The Feel Good Factory

If you expose yourself to negative influences and think negative thoughts all the time, you'll be drastically reducing your chances of success at slimming or anything else. Start by setting up your own Feel Good Factory.

DO THIS NOW!

Feel Good Factory

Make a list of the things that make you feel good. Things that you can call on at any time to lift your mood and give you the energy you need to go on.

These are some examples that people on Lighten Up courses have given us:

- Books
- Children
- Clothes
- Colours
- Exercise
- Family
- Favourite films – you could have your own inspirational video library.
- Friends
- Music – have different music for different purposes, to relax you, energise you and inspire you.
- Particular activities – gardening, dancing, writing, playing cards, yoga
- Pets
- Places (you can visit *anywhere* in your imagination)

Challenge: Setting up your own Feel Good Factory

Make a list in your future Diary of your favourite things that make you feel good, but leave out anything that's outside your control – like the weather or other people's behaviour. Turn to it if you feel the poor exercise and eating habits threatening to return.

Eating

Once you get the hang of Think Before You Eat, and run it every time the Hunger Scale tells you you're hungry, you will find you get more and more pleasure from eating.

Challenge: Enjoying your food

Next time Think Before You Eat comes up with a salad as a menu suggestion, take time to eat it slowly and think about how each separate raw vegetable tastes. Are they nicer with the dressing on? Does it bring out the flavour? Or are some of them better without anything at all?

Variety is the spice of life

You'll give yourself more chances of getting pleasure from food if you give yourself the widest possible choice when you do Think Before You Eat.

Challenge: Foods To Focus On

Be sure to include something from all the sections of Foods To Focus On today.

Exercise

Today while you're exercising, be very aware of how that exercise is making you feel.

Challenge: The Borg Scale

Remember the Borg Scale? When you take your Fat Burning Pills or your Feel Good Exercise today, check where you are on the Borg Scale. Ideally you want be exercising at around 5 on the scale for Fat Jar Fitness, and 6 to 8 for Feel Good Fitness.

We normally use the Borg Scale to monitor Feel Good Fitness, but it's easy to let Fat Jar Fitness slow down to the point where it really falls into the 'pottering about' category. This is just another awareness check to help you monitor your progress.

DAY FIVE

FIRST:

You only have one more day to go after this. Before you start reading through today, write down in your Diary any outstanding questions you still need to answer.

Today's challenges . . .

Motivation

Planning how you'll cope with a difficult situation

Eating

Social Strategies

Exercise

Sociable slimming

Motivation

The Movie

Which was easiest for you? The Movie, or the Future You?

As you now know, Visualisation is an incredibly powerful motivational tool. It's a technique that has made the difference between winning and losing to some of the world's top athletes, but starring in your own Movie in the privacy of your own head is one thing. Living the role in your daily life is something else. For one thing, there are other people around.

The supporting cast

You may have noticed as the weeks have progressed that some of your supporting cast have been less supportive than others.

Some may even be discouraging you from making those positive changes I've been suggesting week by week, because they are used to you being the way you are.

It's understandable. Just imagine how you might feel if somebody close to you started making changes you had no control over, changes which affected the way they looked and the way they felt about themselves. You might be worried that they wouldn't need you any more. Maybe they wouldn't think you were good enough for them. Maybe they would start attracting attention from people with more to offer than you. And maybe you'd start feeling the pressure to sort your own problems out if you didn't have someone to share them with any more…

Coping Under Pressure

Unless you live an extraordinary life, you will always be faced with pressures from time to time.

However, you're in a stronger position now you know what works and what doesn't. You don't have to be perfect – trying to be perfect, like dieting, is likely to trigger failure quite quickly.

But when you're out of your own environment – going on holiday perhaps, at a party, or just visiting friends – and you find yourself in a situation where you're expected to eat and drink far more than you normally would, just pause for a moment. Check the Hunger Scale and Think Before You Eat first and then, if you still want those crisps or that glass of wine, go ahead.

Challenge: Planning how you'll cope with a difficult situation

Think of a situation coming up in the near future that would, in the past, have made it difficult to stick to your healthy eating and exercise plan. Decide in advance what you will do to help yourself cope.

Eating

The Food Profile is a deliberately rough guide to eating. It's not meant to be exact, because the only person who can be precise about what you need to eat is you. There's a lot more to eating than nutrition, which is why I've put the nutritional information separately in Chapter 7.

This much is clear – the one place where it's difficult to remember nutritional advice is in a social situation. However, it doesn't matter whether it's a business situation, a family gathering or a party with friends – if somebody offers you food or drink you neither want nor need, respect yourself by refusing it.

People will offer you food for all sorts of reasons: to show they love you, to cover a gap in the conversation, to make them feel less guilty, or even to sabotage you. None of those is a good enough reason for you to accept.

DO THIS NOW!

Social strategies

Are there situations where I find it particularly difficult to eat like the slim, fit healthy person I am becoming:

- When I'm alone?
- When I'm visiting family?
- When I'm entertaining?
- When I'm at a big party, feeling insecure?
- At work?

What strategies can I use to help me cope?

- Deciding what to eat in advance.
- Eating before I go out.
- Eating slowly, starting last.

- Setting a different Outcome – meeting a certain number of new people perhaps, finding someone with a hobby or a tattoo that matches mine, making someone happy by giving them all my attention, making a new friend.

- Staying away from the food.

- Only having one drink before eating.

- Checking the Hunger Scale and Think Before You Eat and sharing these strategies with someone who's never heard of them before.

Challenge: Social strategies

Design and test your own strategy for coping when you share meals with people you no longer share eating habits with. Write down some poor eating habits and eliminate them today.

Exercise

Joining a team?

You'll make your exercise (and eating) programme a lot easier if you get your family and friends to support the changes you're making. Whether you keep fit with others or on your own, it's important to make exercise an integral part of your everyday life.

On Day One of this week, I asked if your family and friends might get involved in your active leisure pursuits – or if you might join in theirs. Have you worked out whether you could share some Feel Good Fitness or even Fat Jar Fitness with your significant others? But that's fine too – keep going!

Challenge: Sociable slimming

If you haven't done it already, plan to include some other people in your Feel Good Fitness or Fat Jar Fitness programme. It might just be going for an evening walk with your Slimming Buddy, or it might be joining the local line-dancing club. If you prefer exercising on your own, make sure you are doing something you enjoy.

DAY SIX

FIRST: _____

*Have your Diary ready so that, as you read through today, you can fill
in your daily eating and exercise Outcomes.*

Today's challenges . . .

Motivation

Looking to the Future

Eating

Eliminating any remaining poor eating habits

Foods To Focus On

Exercise

Customising the Fat Burning Pyramid

And Finally . . .

Writing yourself a letter

Motivation

Congratulations, you've got to the end of the Lighten Up Four-Week Weight Loss Plan, but remember, you don't have to stop now. The difference with Lighten Up is that it gives you a strategy for the rest of your life.

(DO THIS NOW!)

How Am I Doing?

- Who is responsible for me becoming slimmer?

  _____

- Am I clear about exactly what I want?

  _____

- Can I picture it, hear it and feel it in my mind?

  _____

- How much do I really want to be slimmer?

  _____

- What will I get out of being slimmer?

  _____

- Exactly how will my life be different?

  _____

- How will I feel about myself when it happens?

  _____

- How strong is my belief that I will be slimmer?

  _____ ⇨

- What evidence do I have for it?

  _____

- Am I ready and willing to continue taking action?

  _____

- What could I do to strengthen my belief?

  _____

The Scales

In the past the only scales you've probably used are the weighing scales, to test out your belief in whether or not you were slim enough or getting slimmer. I've suggested you throw them away, because weighing yourself regularly is counter-productive. Weighing yourself regularly supports the negative belief that you are overweight and struggling – otherwise why would you need to keep checking?

If you really do want to know how much progress you've made, look back over the other sort of scales in your Notebook and Diary, and take a look at some other ways of testing out your new belief table and the legs that support it. You'll be able to compare where you are now to when you first started. As you read through the list of ideas and techniques, tick off the ones you are actually using.

1. Motivation Scale

Low   High

1	2	3	4	5	6	7	8	9	10

If you're registering below 8 or 9 on this, pause now and run either the Movie or the Future You. This counts as your first Belief Table Leg.

2. Feel Good Scale

Hopeless		Could Be Better					Very Positive		
1	2	3	4	5	6	7	8	9	10

If you're hovering round 'Could Be Better', take action now. Remember the Feel Good Factory on page 213? Did you make a list of all the things in your life that give you pleasure and make you feel strong and supported? Are there any quick fixes in there that you can use to boost your mood whenever you need it?

What have you been thinking about most, today and every day for the past week? Have these thoughts been helpful and encouraging and optimistic? If not, it's time to call in the thought police and refocus your mind.

Your mood matters because you're more likely to make positive life changes when you're feeling positive and upbeat. When you're depressed and low in energy you're far more likely to skip an exercise session or start eating to cheer yourself up.

3. Visualisation – the Movie and the Future You

Are you visualising what you want several times a day? If you're managing twice a day or more, tick the box. That's Belief Table Leg number three. Visualisation will become part of your life from now on. You can use it to achieve all your goals in life – and don't tell me you can't fit a bit of extra daydreaming into your life.

4. The Food Profile

If you were to fill in the Food Profile for the past couple of days, where would most of the crosses be?

- Are you eating mostly from Foods To Focus On?
- Are you drinking plenty of water?

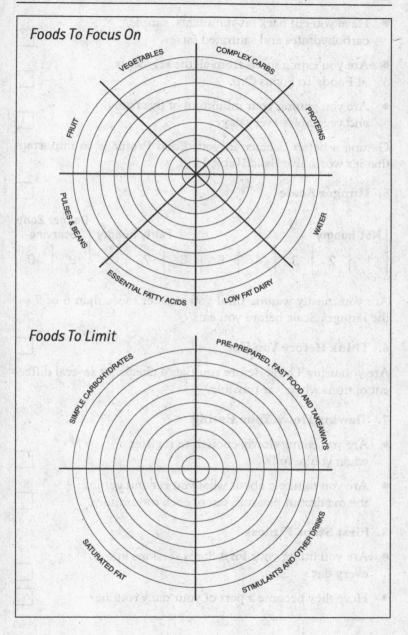

Foods To Focus On

VEGETABLES
COMPLEX CARBS
FRUIT
PROTEINS
PULSES & BEANS
WATER
ESSENTIAL FATTY ACIDS
LOW FAT DAIRY

Foods To Limit

SIMPLE CARBOHYDRATES
PRE-PREPARED, FAST FOOD AND TAKEAWAYS
SATURATED FAT
STIMULANTS AND OTHER DRINKS

- Have you cut back on stimulants, simple carbohydrates and saturated fats? ☐

- Are you eating foods from all the segments of Foods To Focus On? ☐

- Are you getting your minimum of five fruits and vegetables every day? ☐

Getting a better balance in your Food Profile is so important that it's worth five Belief Table Legs.

5. Hunger Scale ☐

Not hungry					Fairly hungry		Danger Zone Starving	
1	2	3	4	5	6	7	8	9	10

Are you mostly waiting until you register more than 6 or 7 on the Hunger Scale before you eat?

6. Think Before You Eat ☐

Are you using Think Before You Eat to check out several different options whenever possible?

7. Slowing Down Your Eating

- Are you eating slowly enough to register when you're full? ☐

- Are you thinking about what you eat and getting the maximum pleasure out of each mouthful? ☐

8. First Steps Fitness

- Are you fitting your First Steps sessions into every day? ☐

- Have they become a part of your daily routine? ☐

9. Fat Jar Fitness

- Are you taking four Fat Burning Pills every day? ☐

- Are you managing to work them into your
  daily routine? ☐

10. Feel Good Fitness

Have you:

- found more than one form of exercise you enjoy? ☐

- fitted it into your existing family life or social
  commitments? ☐

- found time to do it three or four times a week? ☐

11. Outcomes and Goals ☐

Have you got into the habit of setting daily Outcomes for your
exercise and eating programme? Are those daily Outcomes
leading you towards your main goal?

Checking Your Score

How many ticks did you get? If you got fifteen or sixteen ticks,
that's fifteen or sixteen legs to your table and you're doing very
well.

Challenge: Looking to the future

Rewrite your goal in the front of your Diary, even if it hasn't
changed.

Write everything you *didn't* tick as a daily checklist for the
future.

Write everything you *did* tick as a weekly checklist – on
Sundays perhaps – or whichever day happens to suit you. It's a
bit too soon to take those good habits for granted.

Eating

You know what to do now. It's very simple and it doesn't involve weighing and measuring and scientific calculations.

1. Swap your unhealthy eating habits for healthy ones

(DO THIS NOW!)

Make a list of the poor eating habits you haven't tackled yet and how you're going to change them

Habit	What I'm going to do to change it
_____	_____
_____	_____
_____	_____
_____	_____

---

2. Always use the Hunger Scale

You may already be doing this automatically, without even thinking about it. If you aren't quite there yet, keep reminding yourself with notes in your Diary and on your fridge and anywhere else you might need them.

3. Always Think Before You Eat

Like the Hunger Scale, you can soon be running this subconsciously and at high speed whenever you think of eating. Play with it and have fun.

4. Eat mostly Foods To Focus On

Challenge: Eliminating any remaining poor eating habits

Have a look at what you listed in the box above. Kill off those final poor habits today.

Challenge: Foods To Focus On

Over the next week, fix any gaps in your Foods To Focus On and cut back on any segments of your Foods To Limit that are still filling up every day.

Exercise

Exercise Wheel

What does it look like now?

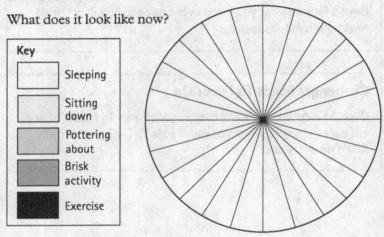

Key

- Sleeping
- Sitting down
- Pottering about
- Brisk activity
- Exercise

(**DO THIS NOW!**)

Debugging Your Exercise Programme

Make a list of the exercise you aren't taking but would like to, and what you're going to do about it:

First Steps Fitness

- How many exercises am I doing?
- If I'm not doing them regularly, what's stopping me?
- How am I going to fix the problem and fit them in?

Fat Jar Fitness

- How many Fat Burning Pills am I taking?
- If I'm not up to four, what's stopping me?
- How am I going to fix the problem and fit in the rest?

Feel Good Fitness

- What are my plans for coping with the kind of problems that might stop me from time to time? For example:
  - lack of time;
  - not enjoying it enough;
  - not having support from family and friends.
- What's my Feel Good Fitness Goal and how am I going to get there?

You can adapt your Fat Burning Pyramid to suit your own lifestyle and mobility. The purpose is to get you moving, regularly and often, as part of your daily routine. For most people it's a radical re-think of both work and leisure patterns, but once established it will keep you fit and active for life.

Challenge: Customising the Fat Burning Pyramid

What are you going to do to your Fat Burning Pyramid so that it works for you in the long term?

If you'd like more information about exercise, take a look at Chapters 5 and 6. They will give you some useful ideas about getting the most out of your activity. There's also a list of the latest bits of kit that make exercise easier and more fun at every level.

Motivation, Eating and Exercise

Putting it all together

(DO THIS NOW!)

Sit down and write yourself a letter

Take your time over this – it's really important

How long is it going to take you to make *all* the changes you
want to make. Eight weeks? Six months? A year perhaps? I'd like
you to write a letter to yourself that you'll receive at the time
you expect to reach your goal.

In the letter, you'll explain to yourself exactly what you did that
made you so much slimmer, fitter and healthier:

- List all the motivational ideas you used – setting yourself
  daily Outcomes and long-term Goals, Visualisation and
  practising Affirmations, and whatever else it was that
  helped you believe you could be slim.

- Make a note of all the techniques that helped you change
  your old eating habits – the Hunger Scale and Think Before
  You Eat will probably be near the top of the list.

- Write down the adjustments you made to your Food Profile.

- Tell yourself all about the First Steps exercises, Fat Jar
  Fitness and maybe even Feel Good Fitness that you made
  part of your daily and weekly routine.

When you've written the letter, put it in an envelope addressed
to you, and write the date you want to receive it in the place
where the stamp should be. Then you can either give it to
your Slimming Buddy to post to you on the right date or,   ⇨

alternatively, send it to Lighten Up, inside another envelope
addressed to us. Our address is at the back of the book and you
only need to stamp the outer envelope. We'll pay the postage
for the one we send back to you.

Challenge: Writing yourself a letter

Have you done it?

If not – go on – do it!

DAY SEVEN

You know by now that there are no new exercises, challenges or targets for Day Seven in the Lighten Up week. You've reached the end of the course! Remember to congratulate yourself on how far you've come in only twenty-eight days. Just imagine what else you can achieve!

If you've arrived at today feeling that you aren't ready, just go right back to where you felt most comfortable and start from there. You can do this at any time you feel you need a top-up in the future as well. But, if you ticked off the fourteen or so legs to your belief table and wrote down your plans for filling in the gaps, move on and read Chapter 4, Lighten Up For Life. Chapters 5 and 6 on Exercise and Chapters 7 and 8 on Food are there for you to dip into whenever you want.

And you can still go back and run through the whole thing again a year or six months from now – if you need to.

You aren't on your own now – you have your Diary, which will be your companion for as long as you want. Take a few minutes to write in it every day and you'll find it incredibly useful and very supportive and motivational. Cultivating the habit of awareness will make it much easier for you to stay in control of your life.

So, good luck again from all of us, and let us know how you're getting on – we're always glad to hear from people who have read the book, so give us a call or write to us. Our phone number and address are at the end of the book.

Chapter 4
Lighten Up for Life

FIRST: _____

Look at the goal statement you wrote on page 42. Decide what Outcome you can set to take you nearer to that goal today and write it in your Diary.

_____

This chapter isn't split into Motivation, Eating and Exercise as you're used to working with these together now.

The Dream Team

On Day Four, Week Three, we talked about your mind and body Dream Team. The *only* way you can be your best for the rest of your life is by opening a dialogue between your mind and your body and keeping it running. The only way to be successfully slimmer, fitter and healthier is to get your body and mind to work together.

The first step is to get your mind in gear – which is exactly what you've been doing over the past four weeks. Your Dream Team is already in training, and you can keep it on top form very simply by taking a little time every day to focus on the following four areas:

- Feelings
- Food
- Fitness
- Fun

Feelings – Your Lighten Up Diary

Keeping a Diary is one of the most useful life-changing tools we know. Your Diary can be your long-term Slimming Buddy.

- When you read back over what you've written over a few days or weeks you'll notice patterns and habits you didn't see before. Once you know what you're doing, you can do something about it, either cranking it up if it's positive for you, or cutting it out if it's negative.

- It will keep you on track over the longer term – plan it out for at least a month ahead with reminders of what you want to do every day and what you want to achieve. Your healthy eating and exercise appointments with yourself are just as important as your appointments with the dentist or hairdresser.

- Use it to write down an Outcome for each day, either first thing in the morning or the night before.

- Check at the end of the day whether you achieved the Outcome you wanted, and, when you did, make a note of it. Also, write down all the other great things you did as well – a long walk at the weekend, or a particularly active day on holiday perhaps.

Over the past four weeks you've got used to making a note of what's happening and planning what you want to change. If you choose to go on doing this it will help and support you for the rest of your life. Sometimes we don't notice things until we write them down. Sometimes we don't find answers until we write down the questions.

Often we don't give our feelings the attention they deserve until we make time and space to put them on paper. Give yourself that time. Nothing deserves your care and attention more than you do. So plan five minutes a day to focus on yourself instead of the TV – or whatever else you'd be spending that time on otherwise.

Food

The next area to consider is, of course, how you're going to maintain your new eating habits for the rest of your life. We've talked a lot of detail on this subject over the past four weeks, but from now on you can keep it quite simple. It all comes down to four questions that you already know how to answer.

The Four Questions

1. Am I hungry?	Check the Hunger Scale
2. How will I feel after I've eaten this food?	Think Before You Eat
3. Is this food doing me good – is it supplying my body with the nourishment it needs to stay strong and healthy?	Which side of the Food Profile am I on? Am I filling in any gaps I may have left in Foods To Focus On lately?
4. Does this food taste wonderful? Am I enjoying this food?	Slow down your eating and take time to really enjoy it.

Fitness

Fitness doesn't mean super-fit and fanatical, but it does mean being as active as possible for the rest of your life. Pills, diets and electrical devices, however well packaged and promoted they may be, are not a substitute for regular exercise. If you've followed the programme for the past four weeks you'll know this by now, but some people still seem to convince themselves that once they lose the weight they can dismantle their Fat Burning Pyramid as well.

At Lighten Up, fitness and slimness usually go together. Being slim for life often means being fit for life too – at whatever level is right for you. But if fitness isn't fun, you aren't going to do it for very long, and you certainly aren't going to keep it up for the rest of your life.

(DO THIS NOW!)

Ask yourself . . .

- Can I imagine what my Fat Burning Pyramid will look like in six months' time or a year's time? The Fat Burning Pyramid isn't a solid structure. It's a virtual one that will change as you and your circumstances change.

- How much easier will it get?

- How much more fun can it be?

Your body was designed for movement and if you honour it, you will reap the benefits. You'll be slimmer, healthier, happier, more energetic and much less likely to eat when you aren't hungry.

Fun

Although there isn't a specific daily Fun section in the course, you've probably noticed our emphasis on feeling good. A lot of overeating and under-exercising happens when we aren't having fun and we aren't feeling good – those poor habits are often a reaction to the pressures of life and I suppose I could have called this section 'coping with stress'.

However, I thought that sounded far too negative. It's focusing on what you don't want, it's like saying 'I must lose weight' and, as you know, negative language isn't going to help you. Positive language is what you need to help you make positive life changes.

Besides which, stress doesn't begin with F and I wanted these four key points to be easy to remember and impossible to forget.

One of the top reasons for giving up exercise programmes and eating when you aren't hungry is stress. Or to put it another way, not having enough fun and relaxation in your life. If the most fun you had today was with a packet of chocolate biscuits (and everybody's had days like that in the past), it's time to take action. If the only way you could relax yesterday evening was with several glasses of wine and a takeaway full of saturated fat and simple carbohydrates, it's time to look for alternatives.

Fun Breaks

Make a conscious decision to laugh more often. Apart from the fact that laughing uses more muscles than frowning, it releases happy chemicals in your brain. Maybe it means reviewing your choice of TV viewing and going for more comedies, or listening to radio programmes and reading books that make you laugh.

Relaxation

You probably know that it's easier to laugh if you're already relaxed. Wouldn't it be great if you could be in a more relaxed state more of the time without food or anything else that's going to harm your health?

The simplest thing you can do to reduce your stress levels is to pay more attention to your breathing as well as to your eating and exercise.

So, stop for a moment now, and for the next five breaths count yourself in and out. Breathe in to a count of ten and then breathe out again to a count of ten. If breathing is something you take for granted, you'll be surprised at the difference it makes.

Learning to breathe like a relaxed and confident person will help you behave like a relaxed and confident person, and it's the simplest habit you could ever learn.

The Feel Good Scale

I've often been asked what feeling good has got to do with slimming.

'Why do you eat when you aren't hungry?' I ask.

'It makes me feel better,' is the usual answer.

Food is only a short-term remedy. Eating is for pleasure and hunger, but, when it comes to having fun, there are more direct ways of doing it that don't make you fat. You've already written down some of them and you can make some space in your Diary to add to that list and build up your own library of personal resources.

Remember, fun often goes with music and physical activity. Some of your fun resources might well involve either Fat Jar Fitness or Feel Good Fitness.

And that is just about it. Simple, isn't it? All you have to do from now on is remember the four Fs and promise yourself you're going to be slimmer, fitter and more fun in future.

If you'd like some support . . .

You can check out Chapters 5, 6, 7 and 8 for more information on eating and exercise (or Food and Fitness if you prefer) and start back at the beginning, or any other point, of the Lighten Up Four-Week Weight Loss Plan any time you feel like a refresher course. There are audiotapes available to help you with the Visualisation and if you need a bit more inspiration we have one-day workshops as well as live courses across the UK. Our address and phone number are at the end of the book if you'd like to know more.

So, good luck from all of us at Lighten Up and remember to give us a call if you have any queries or if you want to tell us how well you're doing. We'd love to hear from you.

Chapter 5

Exercise

The Fat Burning Pyramid

Good news about exercise

Most people will do anything to avoid exercising. We will diet to within a calorie of our daily needs rather than walk up an escalator, but exercise is just as important as a healthy diet when it comes to staying slim. If you're really serious about getting slimmer and staying slimmer, you have no choice. Exercise isn't just an option, it's the only way.

For a lot of people that's bad news and they just don't want to hear it. However, the good news is that once you start exercising regularly – at whatever level you can manage – you will start to enjoy it.

In 1995, the Health Education Authority Report* stated that exercise is a very important factor in managing obesity. They also stated that it would greatly reduce diabetes, coronary heart disease, cancer and osteoporosis, and that it was even helpful to people suffering from depression.

The recommended exercise levels weren't very strenuous:

- at least 30 minutes of moderate intensity activity on at least five days a week to achieve health benefits and to reduce mortality (Fat Jar Fitness);

*The Health Education Authority became the Health Development Agency in 2000.

- at least 20 minutes of vigorous intensity activity on three or more days a week, which increases aerobic fitness and reduces mortality (Feel Good Fitness).

I'm suggesting you do a bit more than the Department of Health-recommended minimums because you want to be better than just average, don't you?

Feel Good Fitness

In order to qualify as Feel Good Fitness any form of cardiovascular exercise should take you up to 7 or 8 on the Borg Scale and, if you want to know what that is in terms of your pulse rate, the easy way is to subtract your age from 220 and then work to about 65–80% of that. If you are forty, for example, you would be working at 65–80% of 180 which would be a pulse rate of between 117 and 144 per minute.

Ideally, Feel Good Fitness includes a combination of aerobic activity and resistance training or toning exercises.

Signs that you're working at Feel Good Fitness level

- You can talk at the same time, but if you're breathing between each word you're working too hard. On the other hand, if you're talking normally you need to speed up.

- Breathing faster.

- You're in a rhythm and, although you're breathing hard, you feel as though you can last for a long time.

Signs that you may be pushing yourself too hard

- Panting is usually shallow and you may start gasping for breath.

- If you start to labour, or lose your rhythm or you suddenly feel it's getting much harder.

- If you start to feel pain *anywhere*, stop. Remember the location of the pain is not necessarily the source – pain in your legs, for example, may be to do with your back. Walk, stretch and move around until you get a fix on how you really feel.

Get to know what's right for you.

The Top Ten Feel Good Fitness Questions

Feel Good Fitness can be a highly technical subject, and if you really want to get into it in a big way, you need to join a club and take advice directly from a qualified personal trainer. However, if you just want to get moving and keep fit at a slightly more strenuous level than the Fat Jar, here are the simple answers to the top ten questions that Lighten Up course members regularly ask.

What do I need to know about:

1. Aerobic exercise?
2. Fat burning and afterburning?
3. Fitness clubs?
4. FITT principles of training?
5. Flexibility workouts?
6. Metabolism?
7. Resistance training?
8. Toning?
9. Training Effect?
10. Warming-up and cooling-down?

1. Aerobic Exercise

Aerobic or cardiovascular fitness is continuous vigorous exercise such as jogging. It's a measure of the body's ability to utilise oxygen, requiring your heart and blood vessels to pump blood around your body as your respiratory system takes in the necessary oxygen.

It's particularly good for your heart, lungs and of course for the rest of your body! It burns calories and it speeds up your metabolism.

2. Fat Burning and Afterburning

You may be aware of some controversy about whether you burn more fat when you're working at high intensity or low intensity. In fact, you'll burn a higher percentage of fat over carbohydrates in a low intensity workout, but that's no reason to cut out the Feel Good Fitness. The lower the intensity of the workout, the less of anything you'll be burning, and higher intensity exercise is good for your cardiovascular system (see **Aerobic Exercise** above).

Ideally, you need to be working out at all the levels of the Fat Burning Pyramid. The fitter you are overall, the more fat you will be using as an energy source because fat is the body's biggest resource.

Your most efficient fat burners are muscles (see **Resistance Training**, below) because they burn fat even when they aren't being used.

Afterburn happens when you've been working your muscles in **Resistance Training** (see below). The muscles then need to recover for the next session and this recovery process in itself also burns calories (depending on the amount of effort you put into the original workout) and can take up to 72 hours.

3. Fitness Clubs

Lots of people don't want to go to the trouble and expense (and maybe the initial embarrassment) of joining a club. If you happen to be one of them, you can work out perfectly well at home. You could install your own equipment, or make do with baked bean-tin weights. In the checklist at the end of this chapter there's a range of fitness accessories you might consider. Of course, there are also lots of good Feel Food Fitness programmes that you can't do inside a club, even if you wanted to – like hill walking for example.

However, if you've never done any Feel Good Fitness before, or you've had a long gap, it's often a good idea to join a club and work with a personal trainer for a while. You can get professional advice about your current fitness levels, your muscles and how to plan the safest and most effective programme to get you started.

If you do decide to do this, don't just sign on at the nearest fitness centre. They vary a lot, so check out a few of them until you find the one that will suit you best. Here are some criteria to bear in mind:

- Staff qualifications, experience and attitudes.
- Equipment – is it up to date, and well looked after?
- Shower rooms – are they pleasant and clean?
- Is it open at times that are convenient to you?
- Do the other members seem happy and friendly?
- Do they offer a wide variety of activities like aerobics, or yoga?
- Do you like the music? (Yes, it matters!)
- Can you have a free trial visit and join for a trial period?
- Does it have a crèche?

If you do decide to go it alone, there are a lot of Feel Good Fitness options that you can try out at home without investing much time or money. Keep trying them out until you find some you like.

There are also plenty of exercise classes running in schools, colleges and church halls everywhere. You can find them listed in your local paper, shop windows or the library. If you're confident enough, it's best to do these trial sessions on your own. If you go with a friend, or even your Slimming Buddy, their view may prejudice yours and what's right for them won't necessarily be right for you. Join a number of different exercise classes to see if you enjoy them – you'll probably know after one or two sessions whether they are for you or not.

Go to your local library or video store and try out the various exercise videos at home before you commit yourself to buying one or joining a class. At the end of this chapter, you'll find a list of good videos and basic equipment that will help you get started on your Feel Good Fitness programme.

4. FITT Principles of Training

FITT is the simple formula you can use to make sure your Feel Good Fitness is effective.

- **F**requency
- **I**ntensity
- **T**ype
- **T**ime
- **R**ecovery
- **A**dherence

Frequency – *How many times a week are you exercising?*
Twice is the minimum, three times is better.

Intensity – *How hard are you exercising?*
See **Signs that you're working at Feel Good Fitness level** above.

Type – *What sort of exercise are you doing?*
Fun and Variety are the best criteria to apply when it comes to choosing the type of exercise you want to do. ⇨

Time — *How long is each session?*
The usual benchmark is a minimum of twenty minutes for any form of aerobic exercise. But you can start with less and do more as you get fitter – if you want to.

Recovery — *How long do you have to recover between sessions?*
Of course it's possible to over-exercise – but, if you're only doing two or three Feel Good Fitness sessions a week, it's unlikely.

- However few or however many sessions you do in a week, it's best to spread them out as evenly as possible

- Think before you exercise – if your body's telling you to take a little longer between sessions, listen to it.

Adherence — *How are you going to make sure you stick with this exercise programme?*

- Choose something you enjoy.

- Before you start, think about how good you'll feel after the session is finished.

- Visualise how you'll look if you exercise regularly.

- Make Feel Good Fitness a part of your social life.

You can use the FITT principles as the basis for a regular review of your exercise programme, changing one or other of these variables fairly regularly to make sure you stay on track and don't get into a rut. You can alternate between different types and levels of exercise and adjust the intensity of your workouts or the lengths of the sessions so that your body (and your mind) don't get bored.

5. Flexibility Workouts

This means stretching. It's important to include stretching in your Feel Good Fitness sessions.

6. Metabolism

Your metabolism is the total of all the chemical reactions in your body and it's usually measured in terms of the number of calories you're using. During aerobic exercise your metabolic rate will increase dramatically and you'll be burning more calories, some of which will be fat and some will be carbohydrates (see **Fat Burning and Afterburning** above).

7. Resistance Training

Also known as weight training, it means flexing your muscles against some resistance in order to make them stronger. There are lots of good reasons to do it:

- It builds muscles which are great fat burners – this is why resistance training is very important to successful slimming.

- It makes you look good. You'll look defined rather than flabby.

- It increases bone density to help prevent osteoporosis (the best prevention for osteoporosis is weight bearing exercise, i.e. aerobics/running etc.).

- It works on specific parts of your body – there's no such thing as spot fat reduction but you can work on particular muscles.

Most forms of exercise have an element of resistance in them – after all, if you run, you are pushing your leg muscles against the ground, and with swimming you're getting resistance from the water – but if you want to start weight training for the first time, it's best to take professional advice so that you do it correctly and don't risk straining or injuring yourself.

Resistance training terminology:

- Form – the correct technique – is important, and deviating from it is one of the main causes of injury.

- Repetition – this simply means lifting the weight and lowering it again once.

- Set – this is a particular number of repetitions with a particular resistance weight.

- Time – setting a time for each repetition helps maintain your technique (you'll notice yourself speeding up as you get tired).

8. Toning

The more muscle you have, the higher your resting metabolic rate will be – this is why resistance training is more accurately called body *toning* rather than body *building*.

In Chapter 6 you'll find the Lighten Up Home Exercise Programme which provides a good basic resistance/toning workout you can do at home.

9. The Training Effect

This is what happens when your Feel Good Fitness programme gets a bit too easy and comfortable. However, you don't need constantly to increase your time and intensity in order to avoid the Training Effect.

All that's needed is variety. Of course, at the beginning you can increase the length of your Feel Good session or the size of the weights you're lifting, but you can also introduce different kinds of exercise, working different muscles in a variety of different activities.

10. Warming-Up And Cooling-Down

Whatever Feel Good Fitness you do will put a strain on your muscles, so it's important to give yourself time at the beginning and end of your session to warm-up and cool-down. It's important that before you start to put any strain on your muscles they are actually a degree or so warmer than their resting temperature would be.

- Warm-up slowly, taking about five minutes to build up to the speed and intensity of exercise you're aiming to settle at.

- Cool-down for about the same length of time, gradually slowing down until your breathing is back to normal.

Allow yourself some leeway on the timing – if you've just got out of bed, or you're tired and your joints are stiff, take a bit longer to warm-up. The same goes for the cool-down. If you've been working harder or for longer than usual, give yourself longer to cool down.

Fat Jar Fitness

Where does Fat Jar Fitness fit into all of this? Fat Jar Fitness is your baseline activity that decides whether or not you stay permanently slim, fit and healthy. Feel Good Fitness is an extra, bonus level of fitness.

If you build regular activity into your life by walking and cycling, using your car less and putting a bit more oomph into routine tasks like cleaning and gardening, you'll also get greater benefit from your Feel Good Fitness sessions. For a start, those activities will be more likely to energise you than tire you out if you do them that way.

What do you need?

The only real requirement for a regular Fat Jar Fitness programme is a pair of well-cushioned trainers when you're walking on pavements.

First Steps Fitness

The First Steps programme doesn't take up much time in the day, but the benefits you get from it are amazing:

- Like Fat Jar Fitness, it helps you get much more out of your Feel Good Fitness with less risk of injury or demotivation.

- It improves your posture and decreases the risk of back problems.

- It helps you maintain a good steady level of energy – when you feel your first yawn of the day coming on, get up out of your chair and do a First Steps session. You'll forget you ever felt tired and you'll be much less likely to reach for a snack or a stimulant to keep you awake.

Finishing Touches

The first two levels of the Fat Burning Pyramid are free, apart from that pair of trainers. It's also quite possible to have a Feel Good Fitness programme that doesn't cost you very much either – especially if you aren't joining a gym. You certainly don't have to spend a fortune to start with, as long as you have some comfortable, stretchy clothes (and a sports bra if you're a woman).

However, there's a lot of equipment and accessories around which could make your Feel Good Fitness a lot easier and more interesting, so we've put together a basic list to give you some idea of what's available. Most of these bits of kit are relatively inexpensive, but it's still a good idea to have a look and, if possible, try them out before you buy. This is a particularly good idea with the videos – the ones I've listed are currently popular, but you can probably rent them from your local library and see if you like them first.

Videos

Not all of the videos are strictly Feel Good Fitness – Pilates, Callanetics and Yoga, for example, can be used at First Steps or Fat Jar levels of fitness.

Aerobic activity

- *Billy Blanks' Tae-Bo 1: The Future of Fitness* – £12.99
- *Tracey Shaw – Salsacise* – £12.99
- *Tai Chi Chen Style – Paul Lam* – £14.99
- *Ultimate Kick-Thai Boxing* – £13.99

Toning

- *FLOW pilates by Carolan Brown* – £12.99
  Stockist enquiries to 0208 758 0650/ www.flowpilates.com
- *Callanetics* by Callan Pinckney – £10.99
- *Penny Smith's Essential Guide To Yoga* – £12.99
- *Barbara Currie's Yoga* – £10.99
- *Body Control 5 – Powerhouse Pilates With Lynne Robinson* – £12.99

Equipment

Most of these items are available from high street stores as well as on the Internet.

- Ankle & wrist weights, Golds Gym, £8.99 – for resistance training
- Fitness mat, Reebok, £9.99 – for stretches and Yoga, and also for use with toning videos
- Gym ball (sometimes called a stability ball or body ball), Golds Gym, £27.99 – good for strengthening back exercises and resistance
- Hand weights, Nike, £7.99 – good for resistance training
- Fitness Set – adjustable speed rope, folding fitness mat and Stretch and Jump University programming instructions, Reebok – for aerobic fitness, strengthening
- Rebounder – a mini trampoline (increasingly popular for jogging or jumping on the spot and toning leg muscles without putting too much strain on your joints), Reebok, £49.99
- Resistance Tube, Reebok, from £5.95 – for resistance training
- Supaflex X-band, from £10.95 per roll – for resistance training
- Skipping rope (you need at least 9 feet of head room *and* floor space so check for space first if you're using it indoors), Reebok, £12.99 – for aerobic fitness
- Step, Reebok, £49.99 – for aerobic fitness
- Total body workout kit, Tricord, £34.99 – for aerobic fitness and resistance training
- Walkman (jog proof CD), Sony, £69.99
- Water bottle
- Well-cushioned jogging shoes (for walking as well as running). You can get away with the cheaper ones if you're just walking in them. However, if you're jogging, then make sure you buy them at a sports shop that specialises in running shoes and will test your footfall to see if you need orthotics (corrective inserts to prevent knee or back damage).

The Last Word

In the end it isn't the clothes and equipment that will make you fitter, slimmer and healthier. It's you, your attitude and determination and, most important of all, your new belief in yourself that will make the difference.

On the other hand, once you've taken that basic Lighten Up message on board, you'll probably find that your values and priorities have drastically changed as well. When you accept that you are well worth the investment, you may find you feel quite differently about spending time and money on an exercise programme that is essentially just for you.

Chapter 6

The Lighten Up Home Exercise Plan

> If you have a medical condition that affects your breathing, circulation or mobility, it is advisable to see your doctor before starting any new exercise or activity.

Welcome to the Lighten Up Home Exercise Plan. It provides a great basic resistance/toning programme covering the major muscle groups, and you only need the most basic equipment:

● Dumb-bells (or small water bottles, filled to a level which is comfortable for you)

● A resistance band

● A mat if you have one – although you can just use a towel

These exercises are designed to complement aerobic work such as walking, running, swimming or cycling.

During this programme, it's very important that you maintain a neutral spine position, as described below in the first exercise.

In several exercises you will also be asked to keep your elbows and knees soft. This means that they are very slightly bent, i.e. not locked.

You will recognise some of the following as things we did during the Four-Week Plan.

1. Getting Ready

Neutral Spine

This is the position at which the spine is in total alignment, avoiding any unnecessary strain.

- Stand sideways in front of a mirror and arch your back as much as you can, sticking out your bottom and chest. Then go to the other extreme and round your shoulders and push your hips forward.

- Now that you've experienced and seen both extremes of posture, find a comfortable middle ground. You should be able to draw an imaginary line between your ear, shoulder, hip, knee and ankle.

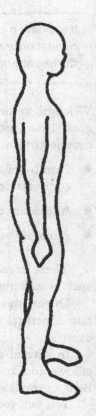

- Keep your eyes looking straight ahead of you and imagine a golden thread is gently pulling you up from the crown of your head, elongating the back of your neck.

- With your hands on your waist, cough. Notice which muscles work involuntarily when you cough. These are the muscles you will be recruiting throughout all these exercises, whether you're standing, lying or sitting, to ensure your posture is correct and your abdominal and back area is strong.

2. Lower Body

i) Squats

- Stand with your feet hip width apart, keeping your knees soft and in line with your toes.

- Lower your bottom as if you're going to sit in a chair, bending your knees to a 90° angle. Keep your weight over your heels and your arms in front of you to counterbalance your body weight.

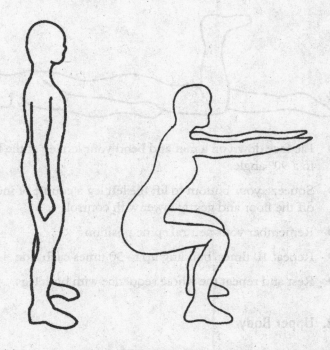

- Return to standing by pushing up through your heels.

- Throughout the movement, keep your stomach 'zipped up', imagining your belly button is being pulled in towards your spine, and keep your knees over your ankles.

- You can begin this exercise by placing a secure chair behind you and lowering yourself to the point where you feel the chair under your bottom and then return to standing. This may make you feel safer until you become more comfortable with the movement.

- Repeat 10–20 times. Have a rest and then repeat the whole sequence.

ii) Bottom Toner

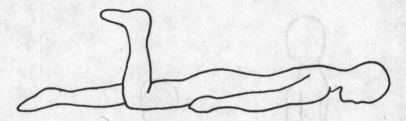

- Lie face down on a mat and bend your left leg at the knee to a 90° angle.

- Squeeze your bottom to lift the left leg a couple of inches off the floor and gently lower with control.

- Remember your neutral spine position.

- Repeat 10 times, building up to 30 times each side.

- Rest and repeat the whole sequence with both legs.

3. Upper Body

i) Press Ups

- Kneel on your hands and knees, placing your hands directly under your shoulders and slightly wider than shoulder width apart. Keep your eyes to the floor, your

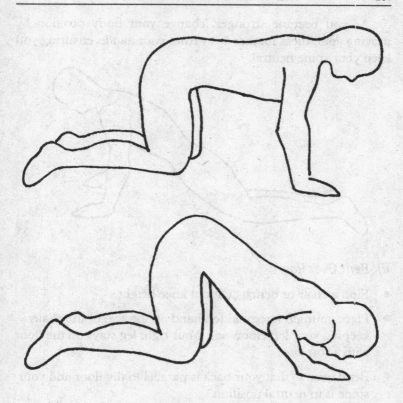

spine neutral and your elbows soft. Bend your arms to lower your body to the floor (or as close as is comfortable), remembering to keep your spine neutral.

● Return to the starting position by pushing up through the palms of your hands.

● Repeat the movement 8–20 times. Rest and repeat sequence.

If you're just starting out, you may begin by performing a press up standing up against a wall. Your arms, head and tummy all keep the same position as before.

As you become stronger, change your body position by moving your knees further away from your hands, ensuring you keep your spine neutral.

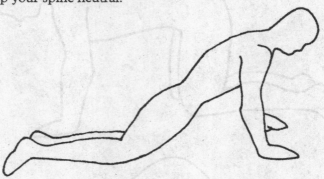

ii) *Bent Over Row*

- Find a chair or bench at about knee height.

- Place your left knee and left hand on the seat of the chair, keeping your left elbow soft. Your right leg stays on the floor with a soft knee.

- Bend over so that your back is parallel to the floor and your spine is in neutral position.

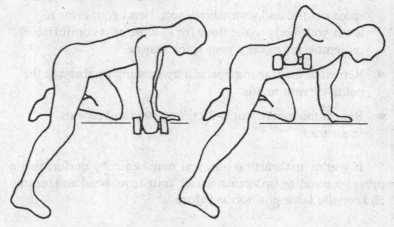

- Holding a dumb-bell or a resistance band in your right hand, pull your arm up as if you're pulling the cord to start a lawn mower. Lower your arm with control back to the starting position.

- Keep the rest of your body still and your right arm should remain close in to your body.

- Repeat 10–20 times, rest, and then repeat with the other arm.

iii) Arm curl

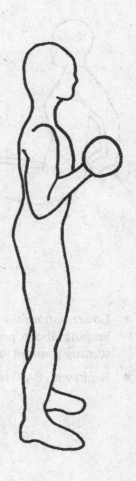

- Stand with neutral spine, and soft knees.

- Holding a dumb-bell in each hand, or a resistance band with your palms facing forward, curl your arms up alternately, keeping your elbows in tight at your waist.

- Keep the rest of your body still.

- Use a weight that feels tough after 12–15 repetitions. Rest and repeat the sequence.

iv) Tricep Dips

- Sitting on a secure chair, place your hands on the edge of the seat, close in to your hips with your fingers pointing forwards. Place your feet far enough away to make an angle of about 100° at the knee.

- Slide your bottom off the front of the chair so your knees are at a 90° angle and let your arms take most of your body weight.

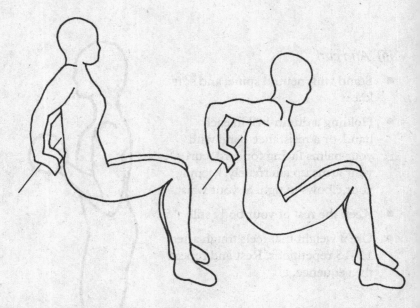

- Lower bottom towards floor by bending arms at the elbow, keeping elbows pointing behind you. Return to your starting position and repeat.

- Begin with 8–10 repetitions. Rest and repeat the sequence.

3. Stomach and Back

i) Stomach Crunches

- Lie on a mat with your feet flat on the floor and your knees bent up. Find your neutral spine position and recruit your 'cough' muscles.

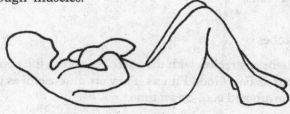

- Place your arms across your chest and contract your stomach muscles to pull your head and shoulders off the floor as far as is comfortable, keeping your stomach muscles as still as possible.

- Lower to the start position with control and repeat 10–20 times. Repeat the sequence after a rest.

ii) Back Extension

- Lie face down on a mat, keeping your arms by your side and your face to the floor (i.e. spine neutral).

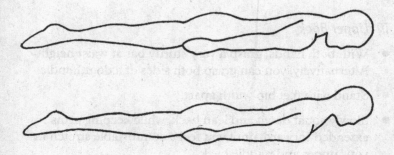

- Lift your head and shoulders a couple of inches off the floor, ensuring your lower body is still. Keep looking at the floor throughout the movement and also concentrate on pulling your tummy in towards your spine.

- Lower to start position and repeat 15–20 times. Repeat after a rest.

4. Stretches

If you do these streches with the exercises above, the combination counts as Feel Good Fitness. They are also useful as part of your warm-up and cool-down time.

i) Chest and Shoulder

- Stand upright with feet hip width apart.

- Clasp your hands behind your back.

- Slowly lift your hands up and away from your body until they have reached the furthest comfortable position.

- Keep your chest out and your chin in without hunching over.

- Once you feel a comfortable stretch in your chest and the front of your shoulders, hold this position for at least 15–30 seconds.

ii) Upper Back

- With both hands, grasp a very sturdy bar at waist height. Alternatively, you can grasp both sides of a door handle.

- Stand with feet hip width apart.

- Slowly squat down and lean back, while keeping arms extended forward, until you feel a comfortable stretch in your upper and middle back.

- Hold in the furthest comfortable position for at least 15–30 seconds.

iii) Tricep (back of arm)

- Stand upright with feet hip width apart.

- Grasp the end of a rope/sock or similar prop with your right hand and raise your arm overhead, with your elbow bent and your upper arm in a vertical position. The rope should be hanging straight down between your shoulder blades.

- Keeping this position, grasp the other end of the rope with your left hand behind your back and slowly pull the rope down.

- Pull the rope down until you feel a comfortable stretch in the back of your right arm.

- Hold this position for at least 15–30 seconds.

- Repeat, stretching the other arm.

iv) Stomach and Lower Back

- Get down on your hands and knees and let your abdomen slowly droop down, allowing your lower back to bend downward and stretch. Hold this position for at least 5–10 seconds.

- Next, slowly arch your back like a cat as much as possible and hold for at least 5–10 seconds.

- Now sit back on your heels with your arms extended out straight. Hold this position for at least 5–10 seconds.

v) Front of Thigh/Quadriceps

Lying down:

- Lie face down on a mat/towel.

- Lift your right leg, drawing your heel towards your buttocks.

- Reach around with your right hand and grasp your foot. Slowly pull downwards, stretching the front of the thigh to the furthest comfortable position.

- Keep your back straight by pulling your stomach muscles in.

- To increase the stretch, push your hip into the mat/towel.

- Hold this position for at least 15–30 seconds.

Standing up:

- Stand on your left leg, with the knee slightly bent. You can hold onto a secure surface/wall.

- Lift your right leg, drawing your heel towards your buttocks.

- Reach around with your right hand and grasp your foot. Slowly pull downwards, stretching the front of the thigh to the furthest comfortable position.

- Keep your back straight by pulling your stomach muscles in.

- To increase the stretch, push your hip forwards.

- Hold this position for at least 15–30 seconds.

vi) Calf

- Put the sole of the top half of your right foot against the wall. Slide your right heel as close towards the wall as possible.

- Slowly lean forward towards the wall stretching your calves. Once you have stretched your calf to the furthest comfortable position, hold for at least 15–30 seconds.

- Switch legs and repeat.

vii) Back of Thigh/Hamstring

- Lie on your back, with your knees bent and feet flat on the floor.

- Raise one leg without lifting your hips from the floor.

- Grasp the leg behind the upper thigh and gently pull it towards you.

- If you are fairly flexible already, grasp the leg around the calf and gently pull it towards the head.

- Remember to keep your hips on the floor.

viii) Back and Shoulder Stretch

- Stand with feet shoulder width apart.

- Link your fingers and push your arms straight out with your palms facing away from you.

- Twist the arms to one side until the stretch is felt on the outside of the shoulder and in the middle of the back.

- Repeat on the other side.

Chapter 7
Food

Food Profile Diagram

A rough guide

The Food Profile isn't split into the usual food groups. It's divided up the way it is simply to help you with the perils and pitfalls of modern living. As I've said before, life is too short to read labels and count calories or grams of fat or protein or anything else. If you follow this rough guide and go for the Foods To Focus On, you'll be eating a healthy diet.

Foods To Focus On

Fruit

Vegetables

Complex Carbohydrates: bread, cereals, grains, potatoes

Protein: lean meat, fish and poultry

Protein: pulses, lentils and beans

Low Fat Dairy: low fat milk, low fat cheese, low fat yoghurt

Water

Make sure you drink at least two litres of water and eat at least five servings of fruit or vegetables every day. Apart from that,

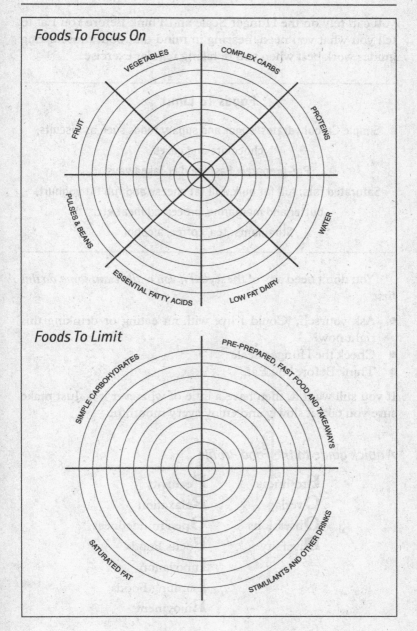

Foods To Focus On

VEGETABLES
COMPLEX CARBS
FRUIT
PROTEINS
PULSES & BEANS
WATER
ESSENTIAL FATTY ACIDS
LOW FAT DAIRY

Foods To Limit

SIMPLE CARBOHYDRATES
PRE-PREPARED, FAST FOOD AND TAKEAWAYS
SATURATED FAT
STIMULANTS AND OTHER DRINKS

you can rely on the Hunger Scale and Think Before You Eat to tell you what you need, bearing in mind that both those eating guides work best when you're taking regular exercise.

Foods To Limit

Simple Carbohydrates: sugar and sugary foods such as biscuits, chocolate and cakes

Pre-prepared, Fast Food & Takeaways

Saturated fats: full fat milk, full fat cheese and full fat yoghurt, butter and margarine, processed meat etc.

Stimulants: tea, coffee, alcohol

You don't need any of these, *but if you really want some, do this first:*

- Ask yourself, 'Could I live without eating or drinking this right now?'
- Check the Hunger Scale
- Think Before You Eat.

If you still want it, then have a little of whatever it is. Just make sure you take it slowly and enjoy every mouthful.

A quick guide to the Food Profile

Freshness   **P**ositivity

Overlap   **R**elaxation

Obsessions   **O**pen mindedness

Diversity   **F**ocus Foods

                       Innovation

                       Limiting Foods

                       Enjoyment

Freshness is a good thing to bear in mind when you're in the supermarket.

Overlap is inevitable with the Food Profile. Some foods are hard to categorise so just keep it as simple as you can. Put your cross in the most obvious category that springs to mind – and if you don't always get it right, it doesn't matter. Over time, your Food Profile will be accurate enough.

Obsessions around food usually spring from years of dieting and working out exactly what you're not allowed to eat. Which is why the Food Profile has been designed to reduce this obsession. If you aren't sure where to put your cross, just go with your first choice.

Diversity is important – how many times have you been told to eat a varied diet? It's easy to get into a rut. If you aim to get a good spread around the Foods To Focus On wheel, you'll be getting the diversity you need to stay healthy.

Positivity about food is unusual among dieters who tend to focus on what they shouldn't eat and that's another reason why Lighten Up is different. We want you to be actively looking for the best possible combination of all the food groups and nutrients you need.

Relaxation is another word you wouldn't normally associate with dieting but the best way to get an accurate reading on the Food Profile is to be relaxed about it.

Open mindedness is the best way to approach Foods To Focus On, especially if you notice some permanently empty spaces in it. People can be very rigid about what they will and won't eat and that seriously limits their options for staying slim, fit and healthy. Experiment with Foods To Focus On that you haven't tried yet.

Focus Foods are listed later on in the chapter, so if you still aren't sure where to put your tuna sandwich on brown*, that's where you can find out.

Innovation will make it easier for you to change your eating habits. Healthy eating needn't be boring, so check the recipes in Chapter 8 and start experimenting.

Limiting Foods are probably easier to recognise than Focus Foods, but I've listed them anyway.

Enjoyment is the key to success. Getting the maximum pleasure from your new eating pattern will help you stick to it. Eat slowly and really, really enjoy.

The Food Lists

We can't list everything – it would take up the whole book. The commonest foods are here, but if you have any particularly unusual food preferences and you really can't work it out, by all means, give us a call.

There are no serving sizes because I assume that the sizes of the human beings reading this book will vary quite a bit. If you are a six-foot, twenty-year-old male with an active job, your food requirements are going to be much higher than a five-foot, fifty-year-old female sitting at a desk all day. One way of judging portion size is to think of a serving as a small handful, assuming the size of your hand corresponds to the size of your body.

However, the best way is to use the step-by-step guide:

* The bread is a complex carbohydrate and the tuna is both protein and essential fatty acids – see what I mean about not being too precise?

Personalised Portion Control	
Step One	Use the **Hunger Scale**
Step Two	**Think Before You Eat**
Step Three	**Eat slowly**
Step Four	**Stop** when you're full
Result	You'll probably find you consumed exactly what you needed

Foods To Focus On

Fruit

Apples
Apricots
Bananas
Berries
Cherries
Dried fruit
  (not processed or sugared)
Figs
Grapefruit
Grapes

Kiwis
Lemons
Mangoes
Melons
Oranges
Peaches
Pears
Pineapples
Plums
Rhubarb

Fruit contains vitamins (particularly A and C), as well as fibre and minerals. It's a valuable source of antioxidants, which help prevent diseases including cancer and heart disease. It's low fat and it's great for snacks.

Vegetables

Asparagus	Leeks
Aubergines	Salad leaves
Beetroot	Mushrooms
Broccoli	Okra
Brussels sprouts	Onions
Cabbage	Parsley
Carrots	Peas
Cauliflower	Peppers
Celery	Spinach
Courgettes	Sprouted beans
Cucumbers	Swede
Fennel	Sweet corn
Garlic	Tomatoes
Kale	Watercress

Vegetables, like fruit, are incredibly good for us. They contain complex carbohydrates, essential vitamins and minerals, antioxidants and both soluble and insoluble fibre.

They are also low in fat and most of them are low in sugar too, so they are generally good if you want to lose weight.

If you're wondering why I haven't listed the commonest vegetable of all – potatoes – it's because they are also one of our most basic sources of complex carbohydrate so that's where I've listed them, rather than here with the vegetables. Of course there are other very starchy root vegetables, like parsnips, which should be recorded as complex carbohydrates.

A lot of vegetables can be eaten raw or very lightly cooked and that way they retain more of their nutritional value. Obviously there are some that have to be cooked, like turnips, asparagus, lentils and pulses.

Complex Carbohydrates: bread, cereals, grains and potatoes

Barley   Pasta (usually wheat, but it can
Buckwheat   be made out of other grains)
Bulgur   Potatoes and sweet potatoes
Corn   Quinoa
Couscous   Rice: brown, basmati, wild, red
Keniou   Rye
Millet   Spelt
Oats   Wheat
Parsnips

For most people the three main sources of complex carbohydrates are cereals, grains and potatoes.

In their natural, unprocessed, unrefined form, all of the cereals and grains contain a lot of nutrients and fibre as well as carbohydrate, but the process of turning them into white bread,
white rice, pasta and certain breakfast cereals can strip away
some of their nutritional value.

If you want the maximum nutritional benefit from the grains
and cereals you eat, go for the wholemeal, unprocessed versions
and check for what's been added. Beware of 'brown' rice and
'brown' bread that has simply been coloured to fool you, and
look carefully at some of the apparently healthy cereals – particularly high bran ones – that have loads of added sugar.

When it comes to potatoes, it depends entirely on how you
cook them. They contain vitamins and fibre as well as carbohydrate, but they can soak up an awful lot of fat if you deep fry
them.

Protein: lean meat, fish and poultry

Chicken   Lean ham
Turkey   Grilled bacon with the fat
Lean cuts of pork, lamb and beef   removed

Egg white	Shellfish
Fish	Milk and milk products

There are other sources of protein, including pulses, lentils and beans, but I've put them in different categories because the vegetable sources of protein (apart from Soya) are incomplete.

Points to note:

- If you're being strict, take the skin off your chicken and turkey because that's where most of the fat is on those birds.

- Egg white is high in protein but the yolk has a lot of cholesterol.

- All fish are high in protein, but the oily fish also contain essential fatty acids – an extra nutritional benefit.

Protein: pulses, lentils and beans

Baked beans	Lentils (red and brown)
Black eye beans	and lentil flour
Butter beans	Lima beans
Chickpeas	Soya beans
Kidney beans (must be	Split peas
well cooked)	Tofu (which is made out
	of Soya)

Vegetarians can substitute beans, lentils or Soya for meat. Soya beans are a complete vegetable source of protein, and they seem to have other benefits.

Baked beans, which often have a lot of sugar added, are the most popular in this category but there are plenty of alternatives. There are lots of different varieties of tinned beans, which are easier to use than soaking the dried ones. Just check the cans though; baked beans aren't the only ones with added sugar and salt.

Essential Fatty Acids

Oily fish

Oily fish like mackerel, herrings and sardines have the highest concentration of essential fatty acids; tuna, swordfish, salmon, trout, halibut and turbot contain less EFAs.

Linseed oil
Flaxseed oil

Linseed and Flaxseed are cold pressed oils which need to be refrigerated and shouldn't be heated, so cooking with them isn't a good idea. Their structure changes when they are subjected to heat and they turn into a form which the body can't deal with very easily. You may decide that they are more effort than they are worth, but, on the other hand, they are very high in essential fatty acids.

Sunflower oil
Safflower oil
Olive oil
Sesame oil
Borage oil

These oils are fine for cooking, but don't heat them too much or for too long. Their structure changes with heating as well, although not so drastically as linseed and flaxseed oils do.

There are plenty of popular low fat and even no fat foods around, but a lot of the low fat spreads and meals have proved to be less of a simple solution than we all thought they were a few years ago. Many of the low fat spreads, for example, contain trans fatty acids and hydrogenated fatty acids, which are not any better for us than the saturated fat in many foods. Some spreads are better than others, and there are some which actually lower 'bad' cholesterol.

The truth is that we all need some fat, but it's best to go for polyunsaturated or monounsaturated fats in preference to saturated ones. Nuts and seeds are a good source of essential fatty acids and they also contain carbohydrates, protein, vitamins and minerals, although some of them (peanuts and cashews, for example) also contain saturated fat. **Don't** *eat them if you have a nut allergy.*

Almonds	Pumpkin seeds
Avocados	Sesame seeds
Brazils	Sunflower seeds
Hazelnuts	Walnuts

Low Fat Dairy

Low fat cheese
Low fat milk
Cottage cheese
Low fat yoghurt

Both high fat and low fat dairy foods are a good source of vitamin A, vitamin D and calcium, all of which are essential for the development and growth of bones and teeth. By going for the low fat versions you get the benefit but not the saturated fat.

Water

Although everything you drink is mostly water based, it's still a good idea to take your daily two litres of it unadulterated. A lot of other drinks contain stuff you just don't need and many soft drinks, in particular, are full of caffeine and sugar.

Water makes up approximately 55–65% of an adult's body weight. It's essential to digestion and elimination.

Keep sipping and watch out for thirst signals (sometimes we confuse these with hunger): you may be surprised at how much water your body asks for during the course of a day.

Foods To Limit

Simple Carbohydrates: sugar

Biscuits (including most 'healthy' muesli bars)	Puddings and ice cream
	Sugar
Cakes	Soft drinks (cola, fruit flavoured drinks etc.)
Cookies	
Croissants	Sweets
Flapjacks	Syrup
Honey	Tinned fruit (check the labels for added sugar)
Jam, marmalade, lemon curd	
Peanut butter	Waffles

Obesity may not be officially classified as an illness, but it increases the risk of illness and death due to diabetes, heart disease and stroke and has been implicated in some forms of cancer. It is also a risk factor for osteoarthritis and sleep apnoea.

Most of our simple carbohydrates come in a complicated mixture which often includes saturated fats and, in the case of shop-bought cakes and sweets, a lot of other chemicals as well. At first glance a biscuit may look like a complex carbohydrate because of the wheat flour, but if you take into account the sugar and saturated fat, you could probably put two crosses in Foods To Limit as well as the cross in Foods To Focus On.

Pre-Prepared, Fast Foods and Takeaways

Burgers	Indian takeaways
Chinese takeaways (especially the deep fried dishes)	Kebabs
	Microwave meals
Fish & Chips	Pre-prepared meals

All of these are likely to contain more saturated fat, and more hidden sugar than anything you would prepare at home. So, when you're filling in the Food Profile for your takeaway, don't worry about separating out Foods To Focus On from Foods To Limit, even if there is some salad with your kebab. Just put a cross in the Takeaway section. And if you have an ultra size of your chosen meal, put two crosses.

Curries and Chinese style stir-fries are fine in themselves by the way. You can prepare perfectly healthy versions of them at home using fresh ingredients. Unfortunately, however, the take-away versions are likely to be much, much higher in fat and sugar.

Saturated Fats

Coconut milk
Cooking oils other than ones on the Essential Fatty Acids list
Margarine and butter
Most cheeses including feta (unless they are reduced fat)
Peanuts
Processed meat: e.g. sausages, salami
Whole fat and whole cream milk

Stimulants and other drinks

Tea and coffee

These should be taken in moderation because they have a diuretic (water eliminating) effect on the body.

Alcohol

This is probably the biggest health risk of anything you eat or drink, and it's certainly the most fattening – you can consume a lot of calories during an evening at the pub. There is, however, evidence that alcohol (it's not limited to red wine and beer) has some health benefits when consumed within recommended guidelines. Current medical guidelines for alcohol are 14 units per week for women and 21 units per week for men.

Food Supplements

There are so many mineral and vitamin supplements on the market and they are so highly promoted that, even if you're feeling fit and well, you may sometimes wonder if you're missing something. But how on earth do you know what to choose and how much of it you need to take? Should you put together your own cocktail of the stuff or take a multi-vitamin and hope for the best?

Most people with a varied diet with plenty of fresh fruit and vegetables and dairy (by following the Food Profile, for example)probably don't need to take a supplement.

However, supplements are important in some circumstances. For example, calcium supplements may help prevent osteoporosis. If you are unsure about whether a supplement will help you or if you don't eat from all the categories of Foods To Focus On, check with your doctor and see if you need to supplement your diet.

Fibre

Although fibre isn't a food, it is essential to the digestive process. If you follow the Food Profile and eat plenty of fruit, vegetables and complex carbohydrates, you will also get plenty of fibre. The more unrefined grains and wholefoods you eat, the more fibre you will get. These are especially good:

Wholegrain bread, e.g. rye, wholewheat, multigrain
Wholegrain cereals containing bran, oatmeal, barley, granola
Foods made with wholegrain flours such as whole wheat and rye
Wholegrain pasta
Brown rice and wild rice
Fresh fruits and vegetables, especially if eaten with the skin
    where appropriate

Salads made from a variety of raw vegetables
Baked beans and other beans
Lentils, split peas, nuts and seeds
Dried fruit

Be warned though, some high fibre foods, such as nuts, seeds and granola, are also high in fat, sugar and salt and should be eaten in moderation.

Slimming and Nutrition

This is a practical slimming book and the Food Profile is a practical tool to help you to:

● Become more aware of what you eat.

● See where there are gaps and overloads in your eating habits.

● Track the changes as you start to eat a wider range of healthy foods.

I'm assuming you picked up this book because you wanted to be permanently slimmer, fitter and healthier and, if that's the case, this Food Profile has provided enough information about nutrition, without going into a lot of technical details about food groups. We've decided instead to give you some more practical inspiration. Remember, the Four Fs in Chapter 4? One of them was Fun. You can now use the simple, healthy recipes in Chapter 8 to help make the Food Profile more fun. We certainly had fun when we were trying and testing them all and I hope you'll get as much pleasure out of them as we did.

Chapter 8

Lighten Up Recipes

These recipes are designed to help you put your Food Profile into practice and they are based on the same principles as the Lighten Up programme.

They are:

- Simple and quick to prepare.

- Full of fresh ingredients so you'll get your minimum of fruit and vegetables a day. Every meal or snack, from breakfast through to supper, can include some fresh fruit or vegetables.

- Designed to give as much variety and nutritional value as possible.

- Flexible – we don't want you to follow them to the letter or the gram. You can adapt them according to your own taste, adding and omitting ingredients according to Think Before You Eat, and changing the quantities in the dressings and sauces to suit your personal preferences.

The recipes for specific meals are all designed for two people. Just halve them if you're eating alone. The packed lunches are for one.

Sweets and Treats

You'll notice there are no puddings or treats – not because you mustn't eat them, but because I expect you can figure them out for yourself. Once you start checking the Hunger Scale and Think Before You Eat, you'll find your taste for desserts starts to change. For a start, you'll probably stop thinking that sweet equals desirable and you'll start to get a lot more picky. The day you pick up a croissant, for example, take one bite and think 'Why am I bothering to eat greasy, sweetened cotton wool?' you'll probably feel a pang of surprise and regret – but it will make the rare moment when you come across a truly perfect, light and crispy croissant, even more delicious.

Pudding Rules

- Be sure you really want it.
- Eliminate the junk and only eat the very best.

The Recipes

You'll find, as your waistline contracts, that your definition of treats starts to expand. As you're eating more slowly and really enjoying your food, tasting all the flavours and getting to know what you like to eat with what, you'll discover that every meal can be a treat.

The recipes I've included here are all quick, healthy and adaptable – but the main reason I've chosen them is that I think they are absolutely delicious. Your taste won't be the same as mine – but I hope you'll enjoy some of them and that you'll be able to adapt them all so that they become treats for you too.

Compromise Cuisine

These recipes are not compromise cuisine – there are no sugar or fat substitutes or pretend versions of salad dressings and sauces. They don't involve lots of saturated fat or added sugar, and most of the ingredients are from Foods To Focus On, but I've used oil where it's needed and not everything is steamed. It's not standard slimming cookbook stuff and you can make your own decisions about what is good for you and what isn't.

Remember: All the recipes, except for breakfast, are for two people
tbsp = tablespoon; tsp = teaspoon

Unwritten Extras

- Greens – get into the habit of making a bowl of greens part of every meal except breakfast. Of course, there's no reason why you shouldn't eat spinach for breakfast, although most people find, when they first get hungry in the morning, that they want something with a carbohydrate base. However, when it comes to lunch and supper, putting a green salad on the table (the darker green the better) is a very healthy habit to get into.

- Carbohydrate – adding bulk is up to you and your appetite. Often the recipes don't include much in the way of carbohydrate and this is deliberate. You can add rice or noodles or pasta or bread or potatoes according to what you need.

Breakfast

Breakfast basics

Breakfast is the one meal you need never be stuck for because everything you could want (apart from fresh fruit) has a long shelf or fridge life.

- Sliced wholemeal bread (can be frozen so you can use it slice by slice)
- Rolled oats
- Dried fruit

- Nuts
- Long-life semi-skimmed or skimmed milk; unsweetened Soya milk
- Butter

Be cautious with shop-bought cereals (apart from some of the sugar free, natural mueslis) because even the ones which are advertised as healthy often have a lot of added sugar.

Muesli

You can make your own muesli based on health food shop or even supermarket ingredients. Start with the oats and add whatever dried fruit and nuts you fancy. You can make enough for a couple of months at a time and add fresh fruit when you come to eat it.

Here's a recipe for toasted muesli which tastes particularly good.

Toasted Muesli

This keeps in an airtight container for several weeks.

90g rolled oats
15g unprocessed bran
35g dried apricots, finely chopped
20g dried apples, finely chopped
2 tbsp sultanas
1 tbsp honey
1 tbsp water

Mix all the ingredients together, stirring in the honey and water last.

Spread the mixture on a baking sheet and bake in a slow oven for about 45 minutes or until it's toasted.

Serve with semi-skimmed or skimmed milk and fresh fruit.

Toast

There are so many different kinds of fabulous bread in the supermarkets now, and toast is a pretty good option if you use moderate amounts of butter and marmalade. If you have really nice, healthy, wholemeal or mixed seed bread it's surprising how little butter and marmalade you actually need. Or you could try these alternatives:

- A scrape of peanut butter and a sliced banana.

- Beans on toast.

- Grilled bacon sandwich.

- Toasted peach or apricot sandwich with just a sprinkle of unrefined sugar and some seeds scattered on top for a bit of extra crunch.

Cooked Breakfasts

A cooked breakfast doesn't have to be a fry up.

- Eggs are very nutritious – and you don't actually have to throw out the yolks because they are nutritious too, just eat them in moderation because of the high cholesterol content. You can boil or poach your eggs without any extra fat at all, or scramble or fry them with very little.

- Grilled mushrooms and lean bacon with oven-baked hash brown potatoes.

- Porridge.

Breakfast to go

Bananas are particularly nutritious and high in carbohydrate too, but any combination of fruit is great for breakfast. If it's messy, like mangoes or melon, prepare it in advance and take it with you in a box, remembering to take a spoon.

Nuts and raisins – or any dried fruit.

Toasted Muesli, above, can be eaten straight out of a box – it can be a bit sticky, so take a spoon.

There are plenty of cereal bars, but a lot of them are high in both sugar and fat, so read the labels before you choose.

Lunch at Home

Baked Potatoes

2 large potatoes
1 small carrot, finely chopped
75g broccoli, finely chopped
150g low fat ricotta cheese
1 tbsp fresh chives, finely chopped

Wash the potatoes, prick them all over with a skewer and bake in a moderate oven, or until they feel soft.

Cut the tops off, scoop out the middle part of the potato leaving about 1cm on the shell. Put them back into a hot oven for 10 minutes.

Boil the carrot and broccoli briefly, leaving them still quite crisp and drain them. Beat the cheese in a bowl until it's smooth and add the carrot, broccoli, potato middles and chives. Mix it all together, spoon it into the potato and bake it for another ten minutes in a moderate oven.

Veggie Fried Rice

1 clove garlic, crushed
1 tsp finely grated fresh ginger
2 tbsp water
1 medium carrot

½ small red pepper, finely chopped
2 small courgettes, finely chopped
1 cup cooked wholegrain rice
2 tbsp soy sauce
3 spring onions
2 tbsp fresh coriander leaves, finely chopped

Combine garlic, ginger and water in a wok and cook until the ginger is soft. Add the carrot, pepper and courgette and cook for five minutes. Stir in the rest of the ingredients and stir until heated through.

Aubergine and Chickpea Salad

1 aubergine, chopped and sprinkled with salt
1½ tbsp olive oil
2 cloves garlic, sliced
1 tsp ground coriander
½ tsp cardamom seeds
½ tsp ground cinnamon
1 cup cooked chickpeas
2 tbsp parsley, chopped
100g baby spinach leaves

Dressing:
60ml yoghurt
1 tbsp mint, chopped
1 tsp honey
1 tsp ground cumin

Rinse the salted aubergine and dry with kitchen roll.

Heat the oil in a frying pan over a high heat. Add the garlic, coriander, cardamom and cinnamon and cook for 1 minute.

Add the aubergine and cook, stirring for 3 minutes or until golden.

Add the chickpeas and cook for 3 minutes or until heated through. Stir through the parsley and remove the pan from the heat.

Make the dressing by combining the yoghurt, mint, honey and cumin.

Serve the spinach topped by the aubergine and chickpea mixture and drizzled with the dressing.

Sweet Fennel and Pomegranate Salad

2 fennel bulbs
seeds from half a pomegranate
50g bean sprouts
1 yellow pepper, sliced
75g goat's cheese, sliced

Dressing:
1½ tbsp pomegranate juice
2 tbsp balsamic vinegar
cracked black pepper

Mix the salad ingredients. Combine the dressing ingredients and drizzle over the salad.

Grilled Chicken and Fig Salad

1 chicken breast fillet
½ aubergine, sliced
olive oil
4 radicchio leaves
3 figs, halved

Dressing:
80ml lemon juice
1 tbsp honey
1 tbsp marjoram leaves
cracked black pepper

Brush chicken and aubergine with olive oil and grill for 2 minutes each side, or until the chicken is cooked through.

Serve the chicken, sliced up, on the radicchio leaves, topped with the aubergine and figs.

Make the dressing by heating the lemon juice, honey, marjoram and pepper in a small saucepan over low heat and cooking it for 2 minutes or until the mixture is warm. Pour it over the salad.

Baby Spinach and Prosciutto Salad

6 slices prosciutto
3 large tomatoes, halved
olive oil
cracked black pepper
100g baby spinach
100g fresh asparagus, blanched
a few shavings Parmesan

Dressing:
1 tbsp olive oil or flax oil
1 tbsp lemon juice
1 tbsp basil leaves, shredded
½ tsp unrefined brown sugar

Put the prosciutto and tomatoes, cut side up, on a baking dish and sprinkle with olive oil and pepper. Bake at 180°C for 25 minutes or until prosciutto is crisp and tomatoes are soft.

Serve spinach and asparagus topped with tomatoes, prosciutto and Parmesan.

Make the dressing by combining the oil, lemon juice, basil and sugar, and drizzle over salad.

Goat's Cheese Salad

1 tsp cumin seeds
1 clove garlic, crushed
1 tsp fresh ginger, finely grated
1 tsp olive oil
150g red lentils
360ml vegetable or chicken stock
1 tbsp mint, chopped
1 tbsp coriander, chopped
75g baby spinach
50g goat's cheese
cracked black pepper
lime wedges

Fry the cumin seeds, garlic and ginger in the oil over a medium heat for 2 minutes.

Add the lentils and cook for 1 minute.

Add the stock, a little at a time, until the liquid is absorbed. This could take about 20 minutes.

Remove the pan from the heat and stir the mint and coriander though the lentils.

Serve the spinach topped with lentils and goat's cheese, and sprinkled with pepper and slices of lime.

Asian Tuna Salad

175g fresh tuna
1½ tbsp soy sauce
½ tsp wasabi paste (optional)
½ tbsp sake or dry white wine
bunch rocket
75g yellow tomatoes (or red will do)
½ cucumber, chopped

Dressing:
1 tbsp soy sauce
½ tbsp lime juice
1 tsp unrefined brown sugar
1 tsp sesame oil

Chop up the tuna and mix with the soy sauce, wasabi (if you are using it) and sake. Leave it to marinade for 10 minutes.

Arrange the rocket, tomatoes and cucumber on plates and make the dressing by combining the soy sauce, lime juice, sugar and oil.

Fry the tuna over a high heat – for a few minutes if you like it rare, or longer if you prefer it well cooked.

Green Olive and Ruby Grapefruit Salad

125g green olives, stoned
1 ruby grapefruit, sliced
1½ tbsp flat leaf parsley
large handful watercress
45g roasted hazelnuts
½ avocado, chopped
1 tbsp olive oil
cracked black pepper

Put the olives, grapefruit, parsley, watercress, hazelnuts and avocado on a serving plate. Pour over the oil and pepper and leave it to stand for 30 minutes.

Packed Lunches

I'm not a big fan of ready-made sandwiches because, unless you use quite a lot of fat to grease the bread, it tends to go soggy. In fact, this is why we started slapping so much grease on our bread in the first place. So why not keep your sandwich ingredients separate?

The bread is the most important part of the sandwich – and there are a lot of wholegrain breads to choose from, so there's no need to get bored.

The salad tastes crisper if it's packed in a separate container – you can wash it and chop it in advance, so that it's ready to eat.

The filling can be prepared in advance and you can be a lot more creative if you don't have to fit it between the slices of bread. For example:

Curried Tuna
(goes well with light rye bread)

85g tin tuna, drained and mashed
small stick celery, finely chopped
¼ tsp curry powder
½ tbsp fresh parsley, finely chopped
¼ tbsp mayonnaise
1 small tomato, chopped

Mix the tuna, celery, curry powder and parsley and stir in the mayonnaise. Sprinkle tomato on top.

Couscous Tabbouleh
(best with dark rye bread)

1 tbsp couscous
1 tbsp boiling water
¼ cup fresh parsley, finely chopped
1 small tomato, finely chopped
2 spring onions, chopped
½ tbsp fresh mint, finely chopped
½ avocado, chopped with lemon juice

Mix the couscous with the boiling water and cool.

Add the couscous to the parsley, tomato, onion, mint and avocado.

Aubergine Tahini

1 small aubergine
½ tbsp tahini
1 clove garlic, crushed
½ tbsp lemon juice
80g lettuce, coarsely shredded
½ tbsp fresh mint, finely chopped

Halve the aubergine and bake on an oven tray in a moderate oven for about 15–20 minutes or until soft. Cool, remove the skin.

Blend the aubergine with the tahini, garlic and lemon juice.

Top it with the lettuce and mint.

Home Suppers

Chicken Kebabs

2 × 115g chicken breast fillets
1 tbsp light soy sauce
1 tsp olive oil
1 clove garlic, crushed
1 tsp fresh ginger, finely grated
6 small mushrooms, halved
6 cherry tomatoes
1 small green pepper, chopped into large chunks
4 × 50g slices fresh pineapple, cut into chunks

Cut the chicken into 2cm pieces, mix with the soy sauce, oil, garlic and ginger and marinade for an hour or refrigerate overnight.

Thread the chicken, mushrooms, tomatoes, pepper and pine-apple on to skewers (if they are wood, soak them in water for at least an hour before use, so that they won't burn).

Grill gently, basting frequently with marinade on both sides, until tender.

Chicken Stir-Fry with Noodles

250g fresh egg noodles
2 tsp olive oil
160g chicken breast fillet, thinly sliced
5cm piece fresh ginger, cut into thin strips
1 clove garlic, crushed
½ tsp curry powder
1 medium red pepper, thinly sliced
bunch of young pak choi (Chinese cabbage)
250gm baby sweetcorn
3 spring onions
½ tsp cornflour
60 ml water
1 tbsp soy sauce

Cover the noodles with boiling water for 3 minutes, then drain.

Heat the oil in a wok and cook the chicken, ginger, garlic and curry powder until fragrant.

Add the pepper, pak choi and sweetcorn and stir-fry for another 3 minutes.

Add the noodles and onion and stir-fry until heated through.

Blend together the cornflour, water and soy sauce, and stir in. Stir until the mixture boils and thickens.

Salmon Cakes with Yoghurt Pepper Sauce

400g cooked salmon, roughly mashed up
220g mashed potato (roughly 2 medium sized potatoes)
1 small onion, roughly chopped
½ tsp lemon rind, finely grated
1 tbsp fresh chives, finely chopped
1 tsp fresh dill, finely chopped (or ½ tsp dried dill)
1 egg
55g polenta or breadcrumbs

Sauce:
1 large red pepper
60ml herb and garlic dressing
(see **Salad Dressings**)
60 ml low fat plain yoghurt

Mix salmon, potato, onion, lemon rind, chives, dill and egg in a bowl. Shape into eight patties, coat with the polenta or breadcrumbs and refrigerate them for 30 minutes.

Quarter the pepper and take out the seeds and membrane. Cook under the grill or in a very hot oven, skin side up, until the skin blisters and blackens. Cover the pieces in greaseproof paper for five minutes then peel away the skin and chop the flesh. Blend the flesh with the dressing until smooth and then add the yoghurt.

Fry or oven bake the salmon cakes until hot all the way through and lightly browned.

Serve them with the cold sauce.

Chilli Seafood Rice
2 tsp olive oil
1 small, onion, finely chopped
1 clove garlic, crushed
1 tin tomatoes
1 small fresh red chilli, finely chopped
¼ cup red wine
65g raw brown rice, cooked
1 tbsp fresh parsley, finely chopped
1 small red pepper, finely chopped
1 small green pepper, finely chopped
375g white fish fillet, coarsely chopped
125g tin of crab meat, drained
125g scallops

Heat the oil in a large saucepan and fry the onion and garlic until soft.

Add the tomatoes, chilli and wine and bring to the boil. Keep it boiling for about ten minutes, or until the sauce has thickened.

Stir in the cooked rice, add the parsley, peppers and seafood. Gently stir it over the heat for about ten minutes or until the pepper is soft and the seafood is tender.

Salmon with Herb Crumble

2 salmon fillets
½ cup breadcrumbs
1 tbsp lemon juice
1 tbsp fresh parsley, finely chopped
1 tbsp fresh chives, finely chopped
1 clove garlic, crushed

Grill the fish, skin side up for about five minutes.

Mix the breadcrumbs, lemon juice, herbs and garlic.

Turn the fish over and spread with the breadcrumb mixture. Cook for another five minutes, or until it's lightly brown and cooked through.

Lean Lamb and Tomato Casserole

1 tsp olive oil
2 × 200g lean lamb pieces
½ cup red wine
1 large tomato
1 medium carrot
1 tsp orange rind, grated
1 bay leaf
½ tsp dried oregano
1 tsp white wine vinegar
½ chicken stock cube

Heat the olive oil and fry the lamb pieces until golden brown on all sides.

Place in a casserole with all the other ingredients. Cook in a medium oven for about 1½ hours, or until the meat is meltingly tender.

Snacks

Mini Chillies

2 tbsp fresh oregano, finely chopped
80g low fat ricotta
1 small, fresh red chilli, seeded and finely chopped
1 tbsp tomato paste
4 slices wholemeal bread
2 tbsp Parmesan, finely grated
oregano leaves to decorate

Mix together the oregano, ricotta, chilli and tomato paste.

Toast the bread and spread it with the prepared mixture. Sprinkle with Parmesan.

Grill until the cheese melts, and serve decorated with oregano leaves.

Jerusalem Artichoke Hummus
with Rosemary Bruschetta

120g Jerusalem artichokes, scrubbed
60ml semi-skimmed/skimmed milk or Soya milk
½ cup cooked chickpeas
⅓ tsp ground cumin
2 tsp lemon juice
1 small clove garlic, crushed

Rosemary Bruschetta:
4 slices mixed seed bread
a little olive oil
2 sprigs rosemary

Cook the Jerusalem artichokes in a saucepan of boiling water for 5 minutes or so until tender. Drain and blend with milk in a food processor until smooth. Add the chickpeas, cumin, lemon juice and garlic and blend again.

Brush the bread with a little olive oil and sprinkle with rosemary before toasting.

The quickest, easiest and healthiest snacks are of course fruit and crudités on their own. However, if you're entertaining or you want to be a bit fancier than that, there's a lot you can do with dips such as those in the next section.

Chips and Dips

Bagel Chips

4 bagels
3 tsp olive oil
2 cloves of garlic, crushed
½ tsp dried oregano

Cut the bagels into very thin slices and spread them on baking sheets. Brush the topsides with a mixture of oil, garlic and oregano and bake in a low oven for about 15 minutes, or until they are golden brown.

Eat them with one of the following dips.

Salsa Dip

4 medium tomatoes, finely chopped
2 cloves garlic, crushed
1 small onion, thinly sliced
1 tsp paprika
2 tsp tomato paste

Heat all the ingredients in a saucepan, stirring regularly, for about fifteen minutes, or until the onion is soft and the sauce has thickened. Cool before serving.

Baba Ghanoush

2 small aubergines
80ml low fat plain yoghurt
1 tablespoon lemon juice
2 cloves garlic, crushed
1 tsp tahini
1 tsp ground cumin
½ tsp sesame oil
2 tbsp fresh coriander leaves, finely chopped

Halve the aubergines lengthways and bake on a baking sheet in a moderately hot oven for about 35 minutes or until tender. Cool, remove and discard skin.

Blend the aubergine with all the other ingredients until smooth. Cool before serving.

Beetroot Dip

180g cooked, sliced beetroot
60ml low fat plain yoghurt
1 tsp ground coriander
2 tsp ground cumin

Blend all the ingredients until smooth.

Soups

Soups are great because research seems to show that people feel full more quickly when they eat soup, rather than if they eat exactly the same ingredients cooked separately.*

I've included two lentil soup recipes because lots of people tell me they have a gap in their Food Profile at this point. You can experiment with both these recipes and try different kinds of pulses.

Spinach, Lemon and Lentil Soup

120g green lentils
2 tsp olive oil
1 leek, finely chopped
2 cloves garlic, crushed
1 medium potato, peeled and chopped
1 bay leaf
2 sprigs thyme
1 sprig oregano
320ml vegetable stock
600ml water
500g spinach, chopped
65ml lemon juice

Cover the lentils with cold water and stand them for 2 hours. Then drain.

Heat the oil in a large saucepan over medium heat, and fry the leeks and garlic for 6 minutes or until golden. Add the potatoes, bay leaves, thyme, oregano, stock, water and drained lentils and simmer for 40 minutes, or until the lentils are soft.

Add the spinach and lemon juice and cook for 1 minute.

Serve with some interesting bread.

* Study by Elizabeth Bell of the Pennsylvania State University Department of Nutrition, published in the *American Journal of Clinical Nutrition*, 1999.

Vegetable and Lentil Soup

1 tsp olive oil
1 clove garlic, crushed
1 small onion, finely chopped
2 small carrots, finely chopped
2 large sticks celery, finely chopped
100g red lentils
375ml water
375ml chicken stock
1 bay leaf
410g tin tomatoes
2 tsp tomato paste
1 tbsp fresh parsley, finely chopped

Heat the oil in a large saucepan and fry the garlic, onion, carrot and celery gently until the onion is soft (put the lid on the pan to start with until the vegetables create some of their own liquid).

Stir in the lentils, water, stock, bay leaf, tomatoes and tomato paste and bring it to the boil. Simmer, covered for 20 minutes or until the lentils are soft.

Take out the bay leaf and sprinkle with parsley just before serving.

Red Pepper Soup

1 large red pepper, halved
½ tsp olive oil
1 small onion, finely chopped
250ml chicken stock
125ml vegetable juice
250ml water
60ml low fat plain yoghurt
1 tsp fresh chives, chopped

Grill the pepper, skin side up until the skin blisters and peels off.

Heat the oil in a large saucepan and fry the onion and pepper until the onion is soft. Stir in the stock, juice and water. Bring to the boil and simmer, covered, for about 20 minutes or until the pepper is soft.

Blend the mixture until it's smooth and return to the pan to re-heat. Serve the soup drizzled with yoghurt and sprinkled with chives.

Onion and Fennel Soup

1 tsp oil
3 onions, chopped
1 tbsp thyme, chopped
2 tsp rosemary leaves
480ml beef or vegetable stock
240ml water
350g fennel, sliced
Parmesan cheese shavings
cracked black pepper

Heat the oil over a low heat and fry the onions, thyme and rose-mary for ten minutes, or until the onions are soft and well browned.

Add the stock, water and fennel to the pan and simmer for 8 minutes.

Serve topped with Parmesan and pepper.

Salads

A simple green salad goes with almost everything except break-fast (and that may only be a personal opinion). It can be a starter on it's own before a very light meal, and it's good to nibble between courses while you're deciding whether or not you're full.

The salads I've described here are a bit more fancy, but they are really intended to start you thinking about putting together some of your own ideas and being creative with raw vegetables.

Roasted Vegetable Salad

1 small green pepper, cut into thick strips
1 small red pepper, cut into thick strips
1 small yellow pepper, cut into thick strips
1 medium sized onion, cut into wedges
1 medium sized courgette, cut lengthwise into slices
2 small aubergines, cut lengthwise into slices

Roast the vegetables on an oiled baking tin in a moderate oven until they are soft and browned. Check they don't burn.

Mix the roasted vegetables with Balsamic Dressing (see page 311) and leave them to soak up the flavour for a couple of hours or overnight.

Waldorf Salad

Salads don't have to be just vegetables – you can add fruit and nuts too if you like.

2 apples, cored and chopped but not peeled
30ml lemon juice
3 celery sticks, chopped
60g walnuts, coarsely chopped

Mix together and serve with a little mayonnaise. You can use a different dressing if you prefer, but then it won't be a Waldorf salad.

Regular Coleslaw

There are almost infinite possibilities for variations on coleslaw, so try experimenting. This is a standard version, but you can vary the nuts and dried fruit as much as you like.

Small white cabbage, shredded
2 small carrots, grated
½ small onion, finely chopped
1 tbsp raisins
1 tbsp flaked almonds

Mix together – add as much or as little mayonnaise as you want.

Red Cabbage, Apple and Caraway Coleslaw

½ green apple chopped into matchstick size pieces
¼ medium red cabbage, finely shredded
2 tbsp caraway seeds, toasted
2 tsp French mustard
25ml olive oil
½ tbsp raspberry or balsamic vinegar

Mix the apple, cabbage and seeds together. Mix together the mustard, oil and vinegar, and drizzle over.

Greek Salad

100gm black eye beans
½ yellow pepper
2 large tomatoes, chopped
½ medium red onion, finely chopped
60g stoned kalamata olives, thinly sliced
1tbsp fresh parsley, chopped
30ml red wine vinegar
1 small garlic clove, crushed
60ml olive oil

Soak the beans overnight and boil uncovered for 45 minutes, or until tender. Drain and cool.

Cut pepper in two and grill, skin side up, until skin blisters and blackens. Cover in paper for five minutes and then peel away the skin. Cut flesh into thick strips.

Mix the beans with the pepper, tomatoes, onion, olives, parsley, vinegar, garlic and oil.

Jamaican Black Bean Salad

100g dried black beans, soaked overnight and drained
1 medium tomato, finely chopped
2 yellow tomatoes
20g baby spinach leaves, shredded
½ small red onion, finely chopped
1 spring onion, finely chopped

Dressing:
small clove garlic
20ml lime juice
pinch of sugar
½ tbsp white wine vinegar
20ml olive oil
½ tbsp fresh coriander, finely chopped
pinch of cayenne pepper

Cook the beans in a large pan of water, uncovered, for about 45 minutes or until tender.

Mix the cooled beans with the tomatoes, spinach and onions.

Place the first five dressing ingredients in a blender, adding the coriander and pepper after the mixture has started to thicken slightly.

Add the dressing to the salad.

Moroccan Salad

1 small green tomato
1 tsp olive oil
20g butter
1 tsp ground cumin
1 tsp ground coriander
150g couscous
75ml boiling water
25g toasted pine nuts
25g shelled pistachios, toasted and coarsely chopped
½ small red onion, finely chopped
1 tbsp fresh coriander leaves

Cut tomato into wedges and fry in the oil until slightly browned.
Add the butter and cook, stirring until the butter melts. Stir in
the combined spices and cook, stirring, until fragrant. Remove
the tomato wedges and put to one side. Keep the butter mixture.

Mix the couscous with the butter mixture and the boiling water
in a medium heatproof bowl and stand for 5 minutes. Fluff the
couscous with a fork to separate the grains.

Mix all the ingredients together, including the tomato wedges,
just before serving.

French Salad

400g green beans
1 small red onion, finely chopped
1 small clove garlic, crushed
2 tsp French mustard
1 tbsp lemon juice
30ml olive oil
1 tbsp parsley

Top and tail and boil the beans for a minute or two at most. Rinse them immediately in cold water, drain and mix with the onion in a large bowl.

Whisk the remaining ingredients together in a small bowl and pour over the bean mixture. Toss gently to combine.

Salad Dressings

These aren't slimming recipes, but the flavours are good and strong so you don't need much of any of them.

Balsamic Dressing

90ml balsamic vinegar
180ml olive oil
1 tbsp unrefined brown sugar
3 tbsp basil leaves

Heat all the ingredients very gently, allowing the basil to infuse for 5 minutes before straining the mixture into a bottle. It will keep for up to 2 weeks in the fridge.

Vinaigrette

120ml olive or flax oil
120ml white wine vinegar
cracked black pepper
sea salt
2 tbsp wholegrain mustard

Whisk all the ingredients together. They will separate again, but you can shake them to recombine them. Store in the fridge for up to 3 weeks.

Herb and Garlic Dressing

Follow the recipe for the Vinaigrette dressing adding:

1 clove garlic, crushed
3 tbsp basil or coriander leaves
(or any other herb you wish to use)

Thai Dressing

1 tbsp sesame oil
80ml light soy sauce
2 tbsp lime juice
1 tbsp unrefined brown sugar
2 red chillies, chopped

Mix all the ingredients and store it in the fridge for up to a week.

Eating Out

Rules for Eating Out

- Eating in restaurants is the perfect opportunity to run Think Before You Eat with some genuine choices. Take your time.

- If you eat out rarely, take your time and enjoy. It's a chance to eat really slowly – after all, you're there for the ambience and the conversation as much as the food.

- Pretend you're a food critic and that you'll be writing a report on everything you eat for your newspaper the following morning. Be hypercritical.

- If you eat out a lot, go for the simplest items on the menu, so that you can get a better feel for what you're actually eating.

- Include vegetables, salads and fruit in your choices wherever possible.

- Use restaurant trips as an opportunity to try things you don't normally eat: different kinds of fish perhaps, or exotic vegetables.

- Just because you paid for it doesn't mean you have to eat it all. Food may be wasted in the restaurant bin, but if you put it inside you when you aren't hungry, it's worse than wasted because it's adding fat to your body.

- If you can drive through it or take it away, it probably isn't good for you (although there are exceptions to this – these days there are more healthy take-away options such as sushi and salad etc).

Chapter 9

Troubleshooting

The courses we run come complete with a personal trainer for people to turn to if they get a bit stuck, but with a book it's a bit different. So, in this chapter, we've included ten of the most frequently asked questions – and answers which might help you if you need a bit of support.

1. What If . . . I'm not sure I'm going to have time to Lighten Up?

If you're asking yourself, 'How am I going to find the time to read through all this and squeeze in exercise sessions as well?' then here's something to think about.

Being overweight, unhealthy and unhappy is much more time consuming in the long run than the things I'll be asking you to do. As you read the book, you'll start to notice how much time you spend every day doing things that don't get you anywhere and don't make you happy either: lying in bed feeling bad about yourself, for example – instead of constructively visualising yourself looking good.

I'm amazed at how many people tell me they don't have a minute to spare, and then manage eight or nine cigarette breaks (at least five minutes each) every day. That's more than enough time for a First Steps session.

OK, you may not be a smoker, but we all have our self-destructive habits that eat up little bits of time here and there.

What's to stop you from using those same little bits of bad habit time to make you feel good and start slimming?

2. What If . . . I'm trying to use the Hunger Scale but I'm feeling hungry all the time?

There are five main reasons for distorted Hunger Scale readings:

- A high intake of simple carbohydrates (sugar) can affect your appetite.

- Alcohol and some other drugs will distort your judgement on hunger.

- Thirst is often mistaken for hunger. Drink water first if you're not sure.

- Mistaking some other need (like comfort, sleep, or even exercise) for hunger.

But what if I still don't know when I'm hungry?

- Your body will be giving you signs, but it may be a long time since you listened to them.

- Signs of hunger are different for everyone – it may be just a feeling that you can't describe, but which you come to recognise. Feeling weak, light-headed and unable to think of anything but food – even to the point of smelling it when it isn't there – are all signs of hunger. Start noticing how it feels for you.

- Allow yourself to avoid eating for a few hours, go a little longer than you would normally go without food and notice how your body feels. Pay close attention to the signals your body gives when your stomach is emptier than usual. *Don't do this if you are pregnant or unwell or elderly, or if you have a medical condition such as diabetes. Make sure you drink plenty of water when you aren't eating.*

3. What If . . . I just can't fit any more activity into my life?

Remember the checklist on Day One, Week One? When I asked you about your priorities? Maybe you filled in that checklist and thought, 'Yes! My health has to be more of a priority for me – after all, I owe it to myself/my family/my friends to stay in shape.'

And now, just a few days later, you're frustrated because it's still as difficult as it ever was to find the time to fit in your fifteen-minute Fat Burning Pills, let alone anything else.

It could be that you're still working on the all or nothing principle which has ruled slimming programmes for so long. You know what I mean – you swing between total abstinence and eating everything in sight, you work out every day until you injure yourself, and then you go back to driving to the corner shop because five minutes seems too far to walk. That kind of thinking is a fast route to failure.

Life doesn't work like that and neither does Lighten Up. If you want to change the habits of a lifetime, you've got a better chance if you chip away at it: eating the elephant a bite at a time.

If you can't take fifteen-minute Fat Jar Fitness breaks in one go, why not start with five minutes every hour? It's still a Fat Burning Pill – just a lower dose. Most of us, whether we're operating a computer, a kitchen sink, a baby buggy or a forklift truck, can take a break every hour or so. Just make it brisk.

Have a break, have a Fat Jar Break

Think of the breaks you take already. What do you do with them? Are you one of the smokers outside the city office blocks? One of the queue at the bus stop? Sitting at the kitchen table with a cup of coffee because you have a spare five minutes? Isn't it odd that, in a society where most of us use our brains more than our bodies, taking a break means physically doing even less than we were doing before?

Just suppose you could re-define taking a break as taking a Fat Burning Pill instead and getting up and going for a walk?

4. What If . . . The idea of being allowed to eat anything I like is too scary and I'm afraid of losing control of my eating altogether?

- Your experience has probably taught you to be afraid – especially if you've dieted in the past. The message most slimming programmes give is that, left to yourself, you'd eat uncontrollably – you may even have done that in the past – but you can change both the belief and the behaviour.

- If you listen to your body, you'll gradually realise that it only asks for as much food as it needs. But if you listen to your mind, you may get requests for excess food to meet emotional needs.

You have a choice – you can go on being afraid, or you can take a risk and trust your body. What have you got to lose (other than weight of course)? Your previous methods obviously didn't work – and if this one doesn't, you can always go back to behaving as if food is not your friend.

5. What If . . . I just can't visualise?

- When you're doing The Future You – or any Visualisation exercise – look upwards and relax. When we daydream we usually look up, as if we were looking at pictures in our heads, and if you start by shifting your gaze upwards you make the process easier.

- Remember when we did the Scrooge exercise at the beginning? I suspect you found it easy enough to imagine yourself gaining weight, getting tired, unfit and out of breath and wearing baggier clothes. Most of us picture disasters more easily than triumphs, yet the mental process is exactly the same.

- And can you remember the last food you ate? What it looked like, smelled like and tasted like? Can you imagine the meal you'd like to eat next? Your brain doesn't know the difference between the meal you just ate and the one you didn't. There's no reason why you can't imagine something you want just as easily as picturing reality – if I ask you to picture a blue elephant, you'll probably be able to do it, so you can also picture the slim, healthy you.

- Some people find it easier to get a feel for things, or hear comments about things rather than picturing them. If you're one of those people, an important part of visualisation for you will be getting into how you'll feel at your ideal weight, or you might hear people talking about you. Most people think in pictures, but if you rely more on your other senses, by all means use them to get that image you want of yourself when you're slimmer, fitter and healthier.

6. What If . . . I still can't imagine myself enjoying exercise?

- Our bodies are designed to move. If we aren't active enough on a daily basis it's like leaving a bike in the shed and ignoring it – pretty soon it rusts and becomes difficult to ride at all.

- How long have you been thinking you don't enjoy exercise? What made you decide it wasn't fun any more? When you've figured that out, go back a bit further to the times when it was fun – when you were chasing around the playground or dancing through the night, or teaching your kids to swim. Get some good memories and overwrite the negative ones.

- If you can't think of any specific reason why you stopped liking exercise, maybe it's just that you've got into a sedentary habit. It's harder to exercise when you're carrying extra weight, and the less you exercise the more weight you'll carry.

- Start experimenting with as many different kinds of activity as you can think of until you find one that suits you. Ask yourself:

  ○ Do you like exercising in company or do you prefer to be alone?

  ○ Is music important?

  ○ Do you prefer to be outdoors?

  ○ Are you competitive?

  ○ What time of day suits you best?

- Most people who Lighten Up find that pretty soon they are able to exercise at a level that makes them feel good. Exercise is used by some doctors to treat depression and it raises both serotonin and endorphin levels.

7. What If . . . You're telling me to listen to what my body really needs, but all I'm hearing are requests for chocolate?

- There's a difference between wanting and needing. When you were a child you may have been given sweets to comfort you or reward you. As you got older you may have found eating an effective distraction from stress, boredom, loneliness, tiredness and general fed-upness. Your brain has learned to suggest food as a remedy for a whole range of requirements that have nothing to do with hunger.

- Before you learned to eat for non-hunger reasons, you used to stop eating when you were full and you didn't start again till you were hungry. If somebody gave you food you didn't want, you probably spat it out. Until the age of about two, most children are able to regulate how much they eat for themselves. Then they start listening to the adults and stop listening to their stomachs. But the instinct is still there, and we can all tune into it again if we really want to.

- Living on a processed diet with a lot of sugar and salt distorts your instinct for what you need. If your diet is high in simple carbohydrates it may be a little more difficult to get a true reading from the Think Before You Eat exercise – more difficult, but still possible!

- Not getting enough exercise may mean you don't have enough dopamine receptors to regulate your appetite. Regular exercise makes it much easier to know whether you're truly hungry or not.*

8. What If . . . I still don't believe it's possible for me to stay slim permanently?

- You will be able to see it more clearly when you believe it (not vice versa as commonly believed). So the real question is: 'How can I change that negative belief?'

- In your Diary draw up two columns. One column is for all the reasons that support the old negative belief and the other column is for all the reasons that might make you believe you can be slim. It would look like the one illustrated opposite (I've suggested some reasons, and left room for you to add others):

Reasons why I'll always be overweight	Reasons why I can be permanently slim
• I always put weight back on when I've lost it before	• I'm using the Hunger Scale
• I still eat too many cakes, crisps and confectionery	• I'm exercising regularly 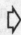

* Brookhaven National Laboratory, New York 2001.

Reasons why I'll always be overweight	Reasons why I can be permanently slim
• My lifestyle makes it difficult to eat healthy food	• I'm walking to work
• I still haven't got time to exercise	• I'm eating more fruit and vegetables
• _____	• _____
• _____	• _____
• _____	• _____
• _____	• _____

9. What If . . . My family and friends aren't giving me as much encouragement as I expected?

It doesn't matter if the very people who encouraged you to try Lighten Up are now buying you sweets and offering you cake. They may just feel a bit anxious as you start to change. They're used to you being the way you are – or were. It may help if you explain to them how you feel when they press you to eat food you don't want. But the truth is that you don't need anyone's permission to do this. It's for you.

So, go ahead. They'll come on board once they realise how much better it's making you feel about yourself.

10. What If . . . I'm not sure I'll remember all this when I don't have the daily reminders?

All the ideas and techniques I've been giving you are aimed at making you self-sufficient for life. That's why you don't have a diet sheet or a calorie allowance – or even a specific exercise programme. The reason other slimming programmes may have failed you in the past is that many of them are designed to make you dependent on a particular system rather than being self-reliant.

If you're still feeling a bit uncertain, here are some reasons why you needn't be:

- The Success Formula can be applied at any time if you start to feel out of control.

- If you're knocked off course by pressure, overwork, illness or other people, remember it's just a lapse. You can always run through the programme again at any time, starting from the beginning or at any point you choose. It's always there for you.

- If you'd like a bit more help to focus you on some of the visualisation techniques, there are two Lighten Up tapes which you can keep in your car or kitchen or lounge or bedroom and listen to whenever you have a free moment.*

- If you've been doing this with a Slimming Buddy, make arrangements to meet regularly for follow-up sessions, so that you can support each other. You needn't struggle with this alone if you take steps to build up a support network.

* *Lighten Up*, published by Random House Audiobooks; *Slimming With Pete*, available from www.lightenup.co.uk

Available in Random House Audiobooks

Lighten Up

WRITTEN AND READ BY
PETE COHEN & JUDITH VERITY

**Slimming made simple,
painless and permanent**

The Lighten Up programme deals honestly and
sympathetically with your relationship with food,
it cuts out the obsessive calorie counting and
frantic workouts that make dieting painful and
teaches a new way of eating.

ISBN 1856865452

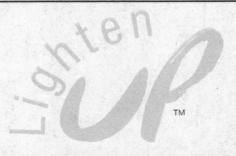

A range of Lighten Up courses and products are now available. To receive your free information pack

call us on **0845 603 3456**
(calls charged at local rate)

visit us at **www.lightenup@bupa.com**

email us at **info@lightenup.co.uk**

or return the slip below to

**Lighten Up Ltd
Ash House Littleton Road Ashford
Twickenham TW15 1TZ**

PLEASE SEND A FREE INFORMATION PACK TO:

Title: _____ First name: _____ Surname: _____

Address: _____

_____

_____

Postcode: _____

Home phone: _____

email address: _____